ORL

OXFORD RHEUMATOLOGY LIBRARY

Myositis

O R L

OXFORD RHEUMATOLOGY LIBRARY

Myositis

Edited by

Hector Chinoy

Senior Lecturer in Rheumatology, NIHR Manchester Biomedical
Research Centre, Central Manchester University Hospitals NHS
Foundation Trust, Manchester Academic Health Science Centre,
University of Manchester, UK

Robert G Cooper

Professor of Medicine (Muscle & Rheumatology), MRC/ARUK
Centre for Integrated Research into Musculoskeletal Ageing,
University of Liverpool, UK

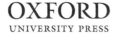

OXFORD
UNIVERSITY PRESS

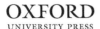

OXFORD
UNIVERSITY PRESS

Great Clarendon Street, Oxford, OX2 6DP,
United Kingdom

Oxford University Press is a department of the University of Oxford.
It furthers the University's objective of excellence in research, scholarship,
and education by publishing worldwide. Oxford is a registered trade mark of
Oxford University Press in the UK and in certain other countries

First Edition published in 2018

Impression: 1

Published in the United States of America by Oxford University Press
198 Madison Avenue, New York, NY 10016, United States of America

British Library Cataloguing in Publication Data

Data available

Library of Congress Control Number: 2017954740

ISBN 978-0-19-875412-1

Printed in Great Britain by
Ashford Colour Press Ltd, Gosport, Hampshire

Contents

Abbreviations

6MWT	6-min walk distance test
AAV	adeno-associated virus
ACR	American College of Rheumatology
ActRII	Activin type II receptors
ALT	alanine amino-transferase
ANA	anti-nuclear antibody
ANCA	anti-nuclear cytoplasmic antibody
APMPD	adenosine monophosphate deaminase
ARS	aminoacyl tRNA synthetases
ASS	anti-synthetase syndrome
AST	aspartate aminotransferase
ATP	adenosine triphosphate
AZT	azidothymidine
BMD	Becker muscular dystrophy
CANDLE	chronic atypical neutrophilic dermatosis with lipodystrophy and elevated temperature
CK	creatine kinase
CMAP	compound muscle action potential
CMAS	Childhood Myositis Assessment Scale
CN1A	cytosolic 5'-nucleotidase
COX	c oxidase
CPTII	carnitine palmitoyltransferase II
CRDs	complex repetitive discharges
CT	computed tomography
CTD	connective tissue disease
DAMP	damage associated molecular patterns
DBS	dry blood spot
DM	dermatomyositis
DM1	dystrophy type 1
DM2	dystrophy type 2
DMARDS	disease modifying anti-rheumatic drugs
DMD	Duchenne muscular dystrophy
DOI	definition of improvement
EDMD	Emery-Dreifuss muscular dystrophy
EM	electron microscopy

EMG	electromyogram
ENA	extractable nuclear antigens
ENMC	European Neuromuscular Centre
ER	endoplasmic reticulum
FAOD	fatty acid oxidation disorders
FDG	fluorine-labelled glucose analogue (14)
FDG	fluorodeoxyglucose
FSHD	facioscapulohumeral muscular dystrophy
GSD	glycogen storage disorders
GSD2	Pompe disease
GSD5	McArdle disease
HCQ	hydroxychloroquine
hIBM	hereditary inclusion body myopathy
HLA	Human leucocyte antigen
HMGCR	hydroxymethylglutaryl-coenzyme A reductase
HRCT	high-resolution computed tomography
HRQoL	health-related quality of life
IBM	inclusion body myositis
IBMFRS	IBM functional rating scale
IBMPFD	inclusion body myopathy associated with Paget's disease of the bone and frontotemporal dementia
IFN	interferon
IIM	idiopathic inflammatory myopathies
ILD	interstitial lung disease
IMACS	International Myositis Assessment and Clinical Studies
IMCCP	International Myositis Classification Criteria Project
IMNM	immune-mediated necrotizing myopathy
IRAE	immune-related adverse effects
IVIG	intravenous immunoglobulin
JAK	janus kinase
JDM	juvenile dermatomyositis
LDH	lactate dehydrogenase
LGE	late gadolinium enhancement
LGMD	limb girdle muscular dystrophy
LGMD2I	limb girdle muscular dystrophy type 2I
MAA	myositis-associated antibodies
MAC	membrane attack complex
MADD	myoadenylate deaminase deficiency

MCTD	mixed connective tissue disease
MDI	Myositis Damage Index
MFM	myofibrillar myopathy
MHC	major histocompatibility complex
MMF	mycophenolate mofetil
MMT	manual muscle testing
MRC	Medical Research Council
MRE	MR elastography
MRI	magnetic resonance imaging
MRS	MR spectroscopy
MSA	myositis-specific antibodies
MUAP	motor unit action potential
NCS	nerve conduction studies
NLA	National Lipid Association
NRTIs	nucleoside reverse-transcriptase inhibitors
PAMP	pathogen-associated molecular patterns
PAS	Periodic Acid-Schiff
pDCs	plasmacytoid dendritic cells
PEG	percutaneous endoscopic gastrostomy
PET	positron emission tomography
PM	polymyositis
PRINTO	Paediatric Rheumatology International Trials Organisation
PROMM	proximal myotonic myopathy
PSA	prostate-specific antigen
QMT	quadriceps muscle testing
RA	rheumatoid arthritis
RCT	randomized-controlled trials
RDBPCT	randomised, double blind, placebo controlled IBM trial
RIM	Rituximab In Myositis study
ROS	Reactive oxygen species
SDH	succinate dehydrogenase
SHARE	Single Hub and Access point Paediatric Rheumatology
sIBM	sporadic inclusion body myositis
SMR	standardized mortality ratio
SNAP	sensory nerve action potential
SRP	signal recognition particle
SSc	systemic sclerosis
STIR	short tau inversion recovery

SWAL-QOL	swallowing quality of life survey
TLR	Toll-like receptors
TOR	target of rapamycin
TPMT	thiopurine methyltransferase
UCMD	Ullrich congenital muscular dystrophy
UPS	ubiquitin-proteasome system
UV	ultraviolet
VAS	visual analogue scale
XL	X-linked

Contributors

Prof Eleonora M.A. Aronica

Department of Pathology, Academic Medical Centre, Amsterdam, The Netherlands

Dr Christina. Boros

Department of Rheumatology, Women's and Children's Hospital, Adelaide, AUSTRALIA

Dr Stefen Brady

York Hospital NHS Foundation Trust, UK

Dr Lisa Christopher-Stine

Myositis Center, Johns Hopkins Bayview Medical Center, USA

Prof Marianne de Visser

Department of Neurology, Academic Medical Centre, Amsterdam, The Netherlands

Dr David Hilton-Jones

Nuffield Department of Clinical Neurosciences, University of Oxford, UK

Dr Arash H. Lahouti

Division of Rheumatology, Johns Hopkins University School of Medicine, USA

Dr Janine A. Lamb

Division of Population Health, University of Manchester, UK

Dr James B. Lilleker

Division of Musculoskeletal and Dermatological Science, University of Manchester, UK

Dr Vidya Sadanand Limaye

Rheumatology Department, Royal Adelaide Hospital, Australia

Prof Ingrid E. Lundberg

Rheumatology Unit, Department of Medicine, Solna, Karolinska Institutet, Karolinska University Hospital, Sweden

Dr Pedro M. Machado

MRC Centre for Neuromuscular Diseases, University College London, UK

Dr Andrew L. Mammen

Muscle Disease Unit, Laboratory of Muscle Stem Cells and Gene Regulation, USA

Dr Heřman Mann

Institute of Rheumatology and Department of Rheumatology, 1st Faculty of Medicine, Charles University, Czech Republic

Prof Neil J. McHugh

Department of Pharmacy and Pharmacology, University of Bath, UK

Dr Frederick W. Miller

Environmental Autoimmunity Group, National Institute of Environmental Health Sciences, USA

Dr Jessica R. Nance

Department of Neurology, Johns Hopkins Hospital, USA

Dr K. Nistala

UCL Great Ormond Street Institute of Child Health, University College London, UK

Dr Joanna E. Parkes

Centre for Integrated Genomic Medical Research (CIGMR), Institute of Population Health, UK

Dr Nicolo Pipitone

Unit of Rheumatology, Hospital Arcispedale Santa Maria Nuova, Italy

Dr Ranjit Ramdass

Greater Manchester Neurosciences Centre, Salford Royal Hospital, UK

Dr Lisa G. Rider

Environmental Autoimmunity Group, National Institute of Environmental Health Sciences, USA

Dr Mark E. Roberts

Greater Manchester Neurosciences Unit, Salford Royal NHS Foundation Trust, UK

Dr Simon Rothwell

Division of Musculoskeletal and Dermatological Science, University of Manchester, UK

Prof Jens Schmidt

Neurological University Clinic, Georg-August-University Göttingen, Germany

Dr Albert Selva-O'Callaghan

Systemic Autoimmune Diseases Unit, University Hospital Vall d'Hebron, Spain

Dr Sarah L. Tansley

Department of Pharmacy and Pharmacology, University of Bath, UK

Dr Anna Tjärnlund

Rheumatology Unit, Department of Medicine, Solna, Karolinska Institutet, Sweden

Dr Ernesto Trallero-Araguás

Rheumatology, University Hospital Vall d'Hebron, Spain

Prof Jiří Vencovský

Institute of Rheumatology and Department of Rheumatology, 1st Faculty of Medicine, Charles University, Czech Republic

Prof L. R. Wedderburn

UCL Great Ormond Street Institute of Child Health, University College London, UK and the NIHR Great Ormond Street Hospital Biomedical Research Centre

Overview of myositis

CHAPTER 1

Overview and epidemiology

Vidya Sadanand Limaye

> **KEY POINTS**
>
> • As the idiopathic inflammatory myopathies (IIM) are systemic conditions with effects not limited to the muscles, comprehensive clinical assessment with attention to all organ systems is required.
>
> • Diagnosis is based on a combination of clinical presentation, creatine kinase levels, electromyography, MRI, autoantibody testing, and muscle histopathology.
>
> • Muscle biopsy is useful to make a definitive diagnosis and it also assists in subclassifying disease as dermatomyositis (DM), polymyositis (PM), sporadic inclusion body myositis (sIBM), and immune-mediated necrotizing myopathy (IMNM), each having characteristic histopathological features.
>
> • There is an established association with malignancy in IIM and, hence, treating clinicians need to undertake screening for malignancy and remain vigilant.
>
> • Cardiovascular disease is the leading cause of death in IIM, so comprehensive assessment and management of vascular risks is essential.

Epidemiology of idiopathic inflammatory myopathies

The IIM are a heterogeneous group of systemic autoimmune syndromes with dominant manifestations in skeletal muscle. The best recognized disease subsets are polymyositis (PM), dermatomyositis (DM), sporadic inclusion body myositis (sIBM), and immune-mediated necrotizing myopathy (IMNM). Also included under this broad classification is connective tissue disease-associated myositis, cancer-associated myositis, and childhood myositis.

Epidemiological studies are reliant on the uniform use of accurate diagnostic/classification criteria. Studies of myositis patient cohorts have been notoriously difficult due not only to the rarity of these conditions but also because of lack of uniformly accepted diagnostic criteria by which to select patients for studies. The majority of studies have included patients with definite or probable idiopathic inflammatory myopathies (IIM) as per the Bohan and& Peter criteria (Bohan and Peter 1975; Bohan et al. 1977). These criteria, however, do not distinguish sIBM or IMNM from PM, and they have an inherent potential for disease misclassification. The use of these criteria in some studies, and the use of clinicoserological criteria or immunopathological criteria in others, has contributed to the heterogeneity of populations studied and the consequent difficulty in interpretation of such data.

Incidence of idiopathic inflammatory myopathies

The reported incidence of IIM has varied between 5 and 10×10^{-6} (Dalakas, 1991; Mastaglia and Phillips 2002). A 30-year epidemiological study of 352 patients with histologically confirmed IIM showed that the annual incidence of IIM is increasing in South Australia (95% CI: 7.2–8.9) and this was largely attributed to an increasing annual incidence of sIBM (prevalence of 50.5 cases per million population in 2009, 95% CI: 40.2–62.7; Tan et al. 2013). Indeed, this prevalence of sIBM in South Australia is among the highest reported to date. The increasing incidence of sIBM may be due to increased physician awareness, improvements in ultrastructural examination of muscle, or a genuine increase in incidence.

Gender predilection

All studies published to date have shown a female predominance for DM and PM; one study showed a female:male ratio of 2.75 (33 females, 12 males) in DM and 1.55 (110 females, 71 males) in PM (Tan et al. 2013). Most studies have reported a male predominance for sIBM, although the study by Tan et al. found an almost equal gender ratio (Tan et al. 2013).

Age at onset

For PM and DM there are two peaks of incidence, one in childhood and the other at age 30–50 years. sIBM is the commonest IIM in patients over 50 years of age.

Environmental factors

Spatial clustering of disease in some groups suggests the involvement of environmental agents in disease pathogenesis. Indeed, there have been case reports of a range of infectious agents, including retroviruses, in triggering disease. However, a convincing role for infectious agents in pathogenesis has not been consistently demonstrated.

A worldwide study correlating the prevalence of DM/PM with surface ultraviolet (UV) radiation showed that greater surface UV irradiation increases the proportion of disease which is DM (Okada et al. 2003).

Association with malignancy

Numerous epidemiological studies have convincingly established that there is an increased risk for malignancy in DM, PM, and sIBM, although the reported degree of increased risk has varied. The temporal association between malignancy and IIM in many cases has led to the concept of paraneoplastic myositis and shared immunopathological mechanisms.

The types of malignancy seen in association with IIM are generally commensurate with age and gender. In DM cancers of the ovaries, lung, pancreas, and stomach have been over-represented, while excess non-Hodgkin lymphoma, and cancers of the bladder and lung were observed in PM [Hill et al. 2001].

Recognizing this association with malignancy is of paramount importance in the management of patients with IIM, and treating physicians need to be aware of relevant guidelines for screening.

Survival

Patients with IIM continue to have increased mortality despite the advent of immunosuppressive therapy (Lundberg & Forbess 2008). An investigation into the survival of 370 histologically confirmed DM/PM/sIBM cases revealed a standardized mortality ratio of 1.75 (Limaye et al. 2012). Cardiovascular disease accounted for the commonest cause of death (31%), followed by infections (22%), and malignancy (11%). Risk factors for death were age at time of biopsy (hazard ratio 1.05), ischaemic heart disease [risk ratio (RR) 2.97, $p <$ 0.0001], proximal weakness at diagnosis (RR 1.8, $p = 0.03$), definite diagnosis of IIM per the Bohan & Peter criteria (RR 2.14, $p < 0.0001$), and the absence of autoantibodies (RR 1.9, $p < 0.001$; Limaye et al. 2012).

Clinical features of idiopathic inflammatory myopathies

Effects on skeletal musculature and typical clinical presentation

Polymyositis and dermatomyositis

Both PM and DM are characterized by a painless proximal weakness of the upper and lower limbs, especially affecting the deltoids and hip flexors. The weakness generally develops insidiously over months, although a minority present with rapidly progressive weakness. The pelvic girdle is typically involved before the shoulder girdle. Hip flexor weakness is noticed by patients as difficulty rising from low chairs. Some patients report difficulty climbing stairs or the inability to get up from the floor. Shoulder girdle weakness results in difficulty performing above-head height activities, such as hanging clothes. Weakness of the neck flexors is generally a later development.

Sporadic inclusion body myositis

sIBM has a highly distinctive pattern of muscle involvement that may be asymmetric. Involvement of the quadriceps gives rise to difficulty locking the knees in position while walking and presentation with falls is common. Knee extensor strength is at least as diminished as hip flexor strength and often more severely impaired. Selective involvement of the flexor digitorum profundus with relative sparing of the flexor digitorum superficialis is a characteristic feature of sIBM. Weakness of the finger flexors is often manifest as difficulty pressing spray cans and atrophy of forearm muscles is frequently observed.

Immune-mediated necrotizing myopathy

Patients with IMNM often present with a more definite onset of rapidly progressive weakness. A review of 64 cases with IMNM revealed that, compared with other IIM, patients with IMNM were more frequently male (61%), had a higher incidence of myalgia, and higher median levels of creatine kinase (CK; Ellis et al. 2012). Necrotizing myopathy may be seen in association with malignancy or viral infections, but has recently also been associated with antibodies to signal recognition particle (anti-SRP) and antibodies to hydroxymethylglutaryl-coenzyme A reductase (HMGCR) among patients treated with statins. This latter subset of IMNM has also been called necrotizing autoimmune myopathy and recognition of the underlying role for autoimmunity in this subset provides a rationale for treating with immunomodulatory therapies.

Dysphagia

Involvement of the skeletal muscles in the upper third of the oesophagus and the pharynx may result in dysphagia, which has been reported in PM, DM, and sIBM.

In one study, although dysphagia was identified in 37 of 57 (65%) patients with sIBM on specific questioning, only 17 of these patients had spontaneously reported this symptom (Cox et al. 2009), emphasizing the importance for physicians to specifically enquire about dysphagia. Two questions were identified which correlated the symptoms with signs on fluoroscopic studies, namely, 'Does food get stuck in your throat' and 'Do you have to swallow repeatedly in order to get rid of food?' (Cox et al. 2009). Symptoms related to aspiration, such as coughing and choking may also ensue. Recognizing the association of dysphagia with IIM is important, but other causes of dysphagia should also be considered.

Muscular symptoms that are not typical of myositis

Ocular and facial weakness are not common in the IIM, and so should prompt consideration of alternative diagnoses. Fatigability, i.e. difficulty with repetitive use of muscle groups may be more suggestive of disorders of the neuromuscular junction; similarly, fasciculations should not be attributed to IIM. Episodic weakness or muscle cramps after exercise should lead to consideration of a metabolic myopathy. Moreover, a positive family history for muscle disease may indicate a hereditary muscle disorder, such as muscular dystrophy. Muscle hypertrophy is not a prominent feature of IIM per se. Although myalgia may accompany IIM, focal severe muscle pain is not generally a feature, and this may suggest a focal myositis, localized infection, or muscle infarction.

Cutaneous manifestations of dermatomyositis

In addition to the effects on skeletal muscle, the microangiopathy of DM also gives rise to a range of cutaneous features. Highly pathognomonic for DM are the erythematous papules over the interphalangeal joints, known as Gottron's papules which occur in 60–80% of patients, and the violaceous hue over the upper eyelids (heliotrope rash), which occur in approximately 50%. Cutaneous manifestations less specific for DM include photosensitivity, shawl sign, a V-neck sign, and nailfold capillary changes, including capillary drop out, haemorrhages, and periungual erythema. Gottron's sign refers to erythematous macules or papules over extensor surfaces of joints. Periorbital oedema, facial oedema, and calcinosis may be prominent especially in the juvenile dermatomyositis subset.

In recent years a number of autoantibodies highly specific for DM have been identified and, moreover, these autoantibodies have been associated with distinct cutaneous features, enabling a clinicoserological classification of subsets of DM (see Chapter 12, Laboratory Features).

The clinical correlates of the microangiopathy of DM may not necessarily be manifest in both skeletal muscle and skin in all patients, and may be seen in one system prior to the other. Subsets of DM distinguished by their relative effects on these two organ systems include classic DM (both skin and skeletal muscle effects seen), clinically amyopathic DM (CADM, cutaneous features only with no overt muscle involvement), and DM *sine* dermatitis (skeletal muscle effects without cutaneous signs).

Extramuscular features of IIM

Interstitial lung disease (ILD) is a frequent manifestation of PM/DM and may occur as part of the anti-synthetase syndrome. Dyspnoea and dry cough are the typical symptoms, but many patients are asymptomatic.

Dysphagia is by far the commonest gastrointestinal manifestation of IIM. Intestinal pseudo-obstruction and malabsorption are rare manifestations of IIM.

Raynaud's symptomatology may be seen especially in patients with anti-synthetase syndrome, and in DM the vasculopathy may lead to digital ulcers and periungual changes.

Cardiac involvement in PM/DM is common, frequently asymptomatic, and probably under-recognized. A systematic review of cardiac involvement in DM/PM revealed a range of conduction abnormalities, as well as left ventricular diastolic dysfunction and hyperkinetic left ventricular contraction (Zhang et al. 2012). Congestive heart failure is the most commonly reported cardiac problem in DM/PM. A range of electrocardiographic abnormalities have been reported, including atrial and ventricular arrhythmias, and complete heart block.

Patients with IIM have significantly increased risk of coronary artery disease [pooled odds ratio 2.24 (95% CI: 1.02–4.92)] as determined from a systematic review and meta-analysis (Ungprasert et al. 2014). It is unclear to what extent traditional risk factors contribute to the risk for atherosclerosis over the role of systemic inflammation. Cardiovascular disease is the leading cause of death in patients with IIM (Limaye et al. 2008).

Anti-synthetase syndrome

The aminoacyl tRNA synthetases (ARS) are a group of cytoplasmic enzymes catalysing the binding of amino acids to their cognate tRNA during protein synthesis.

Antibodies directed to eight tRNA synthetases have been recognized (Jo-1, PL7, PL12, OJ, EJ, KS, Zo, and Ha) and these antibodies give rise to a unique constellation of clinical features, including myositis, interstitial lung disease, fever, Raynaud's phenomenon, mechanics' hands, and an arthropathy typically involving subluxations of the distal interphalangeal joint of the thumbs. Collectively, however, the anti-ARS give rise to these features, there are individual differences in relative associations for the various antibodies; antibodies to PL7 are generally associated with milder muscle disease than anti-Jo-1 antibodies, while antibodies to OJ or KS confer a greater risk for ILD than myositis.

Diagnosis of IIM

Skeletal muscle enzymes

Serum CK levels are elevated in the majority of patients with IIM, and may rise 50-fold in DM and PM. Median CK levels tend to be higher in patients with IMNM compared with other IIM (Ellis et al. 2012), while elevations are generally more modest in sIBM. A study of 64 patients investigating the utility of CK measurements in predicting IIM, using muscle biopsy as the gold standard, found CK levels >1000 IU/L had sensitivity 48% (30 out of 66), specificity 94% (87 of 102), and positive likelihood ratio = 8.0. Lowering the threshold of CK elevation to >500 IU/L increased sensitivity to 66% (48 of 83), but reduced specificity to 77% (63 of 91), and was associated with a lower positive likelihood ratio = 2.9 (Cardy & Potter 2007)

Electromyography

Electromyography may show myopathic changes, with a sensitivity of 74% (56 of 92) and specificity of 67% (49 of 84; $n = 50$), against a gold standard of muscle biopsy (Cardy & Potter 2007).

Magnetic resonance imaging

MRI is useful to identify active inflammation, indicated by the presence of myoedema, and to distinguish this from muscle damage, indicated by fatty replacement, fibrosis, atrophy, or calcification. Compared with elevations in CK or myopathic changes on EMG, MRI of the muscles has higher sensitivity [92% (76 of 107)] and specificity [89% (68 of 109)], with a positive likelihood ratio = 8.4, using histological diagnosis of myositis as the gold standard (Cardy & Potter 2007). The imaging of muscles with MRI may also be used to guide muscle biopsy siting to increase positive yield.

Autoantibodies

Identification of myositis-associated antibodies (MAA; directed to Ro52/SSA, U1RNP, and PMSCL) and myositis-specific antibodies (MSA) has advanced the understanding of the immunopathogenesis of the IIM. The strong correlation of various MSA with distinct clinical phenotypes of IIM has enabled these antibodies to be used in disease classification and also in prognostication.

Muscle histopathology

Muscle biopsy is the definitive diagnostic test and useful to distinguish subsets of disease, as DM, PM, sIBM, and IMNM have distinct histopathological features reflecting the differences in underlying immunopathogenesis.

The histopathological features of DM, PM, and sIBM have been elaborately described (Hohlfeld 2002) and are described in more detail in Chapter 13, 'Histopathological features of idiopathic inflammatory myopathies'.

REFERENCES

Bohan A, Peter JB. (1975). Polymyositis and dermatomyositis (first of two parts). *N Engl J Med*; **292**: 344–7.

Bohan A, Peter JB, Bowman RL, Pearson CM. (1977). Computer-assisted analysis of 153 patients with polymyositis and dermatomyositis. *Medicine (Balt)*; **56**: 255–86.

Cardy CM, Potter T. (2007). The predictive value of creatine kinase, EMG and MRI in diagnosing muscle disease. *Rheumatology (Oxf)*; **46**(10): 1617–18.

Cox FM, Verschuuren JJ, Verbist BM, Niks EH, Wintzen AR, Badrising UA. (2009). Detecting dysphagia in inclusion body myositis. *J Neurol*; **256**(12): 2009–13.

Dalakas MC. (1991). Polymyositis, dermatomyositis and inclusion-body myositis. *N Engl J Med*; **325**: 1487–98.

Ellis E, Ann Tan J, Lester S, et al. (2012). Necrotizing myopathy: clinicoserologic associations. *Muscle Nerve*; **45**(2): 189–94.

Hill CL, Zhang Y, Sigurgeirsson B, et al. (2001). Frequency of specific cancer types in dermatomyositis and polymyositis: a population-based study. *Lancet*; **357**: 96–100.

Hohlfeld R. (2002). Polymyositis and dermatomyositis. In: Karpati G (eds) *Structural and molecular basis of skeletal muscle diseases*, pp. 221–7. ISN Neuropath Press, Switzerland: Basle.

Limaye V, Hakendorf P, Woodman RJ, Blumbergs P, Roberts-Thomson P. (2012). Mortality and its predominant causes in a large cohort of patients with biopsy-determined inflammatory myositis. *Intern Med J*; **42**(2): 191–8.

Lundberg IE, Forbess CJ. (2008). Mortality in idiopathic inflammatory myopathies. *Clin Exp Rheumatol*; **26**(Suppl. 51): S109–14.

Mastaglia FL, Phillips BA. (2002). Idiopathic inflammatory myopathies: epidemiology, classification, and diagnostic criteria. *Rheum Dis Clin North Am*; **28**: 723–41.

Okada S, Weatherhead E, Targoff IN, Wesley R, Miller FW; International myositis collaborative study group. (2003). Global surface ultraviolet radiation intensity may modulate the clinical and immunologic expression of autoimmune muscle disease. *Arthritis Rheum*; **48**: 2285–93.

Tan JA, Roberts-Thomson PJ, Blumbergs P, Hakendorf P, Cox SR, Limaye V. (2013). Incidence and prevalence of idiopathic inflammatory myopathies in South Australia: a 30-year epidemiologic study of histology-proven cases. *Int J Rheum Dis*; **16**(3): 331–8.

Ungprasert P, Suksaranjit P, Spanuchart [3], Leeaphorn N, Permpalung N. (2014). Risk of coronary artery disease in patients with idiopathic inflammatory myopathies: a systematic review and meta-analysis of observational studies. *Semin Arthritis Rheum*; **44**(1): 63–7.

Zhang L, Wang GC, Ma L, Zu N. (2012). Cardiac involvement in adult polymyositis or dermatomyositis: a systematic review. *Clin Cardiol*; **35**(11): 686–91.

CHAPTER 2

Diagnostic and classification criteria

Anna Tjärnlund and Ingrid E. Lundberg

KEY POINTS

- Diagnostic criteria are a set of symptoms, signs, and tests used in routine clinical care to aid in the clinical diagnosis of individual patients.

- Classification criteria are a set of disease characteristics used to create well-defined homogenous cohorts of patients for clinical research, including clinical trials.

- New classification criteria for idiopathic inflammatory myopathies (IIM) give a numerical probability of having IIM, and are derived from clinical data from juvenile and adult IIM patients worldwide.

Historic overview of diagnostic and classification criteria

Many rheumatic diseases, including the IIM, are systemic and heterogeneous in their disease manifestations. There is no single test, clinical or laboratory, which can individually determine the diagnosis or classification. Recent advances in the understanding of disease pathogenesis and development of sophisticated techniques for molecular analyses may aid in re-evaluation of existing diagnostic and classification criteria for rheumatic diseases.

Diagnostic criteria are a set of symptoms, signs, and tests which are used in routine clinical care to aid in the clinical diagnosis of individual patients. Classification criteria, on the other hand, are a set of disease characteristics used to create well-defined homogenous cohorts of patients for clinical research, including clinical trials. Classification criteria should have high specificity in order to generate homogenous groups of patients with the same underlying diagnoses, at the expense of decreased sensitivity, leaving these criteria less useful in the clinical care of patients. It is important to remember that statistical performance of diagnostic or classification criteria is greatly dependent on the prevalence of the disease in the patient population under investigation.

Over many decades, several diagnostic and classification criteria for IIM have been proposed (Lundberg et al. 2016). The Bohan and Peter classification criteria

> **Box 2.1** The Bohan and Peter classification criteria for idiopathic inflammatory myopathies (Bohan and Peter 1975)
>
> 1. Symmetric muscle weakness of limb-girdle and anterior neck flexors.
> 2. Muscle biopsy revealing evidence of necrosis of type I and type II fibres, phagocytosis, regeneration with basophilia, large vesicular sarcolemmal nuclei and prominent nucleoli, atrophy in a perifascicular distribution, variation in fibre size, and inflammatory exudates, often perivascular.
> 3. Elevated serum levels of enzymes derived from skeletal muscle.
> 4. Electromyography must show characteristic features.
> 5. Characteristic cutaneous manifestations of dermatomyositis, including heliotrope rash or Gottron's sign.

(Bohan and Peter 1975) were based on case series of patients at a single institution and were developed through clinical observation (Box 2.1). A major difference from the earliest proposed criteria was the requirement of initial exclusion of all other forms of myopathies.

Definite polymyositis (PM) requires four criteria items to be fulfilled, excluding skin rashes, whereas *probable* and *possible* PM requires three or two fulfilled criterions, respectively, with no skin rashes. Dermatomyositis (DM) can be diagnosed in a similar way—three or four criteria items, including skin rashes, for *definite* DM, two criteria items plus skin rashes for *probable* DM, and one criteria item plus skin rashes for *possible* DM. However, the classic DM rash can be so characteristic that clinically amyopathic DM can be diagnosed from the rash alone, when no evidence of myopathy is present. Besides distinction between PM and DM, the Bohan and Peter criteria provided definitions of other forms of IIM— juvenile, overlap, and cancer-associated myositis. Although these criteria provided major advantages over the previous attempts, several limitations have been identified. Apart from being empirically derived they do not provide definitions on the criteria items, such as the characteristic features of DM or how to rule out other forms of myopathies, leaving these features to be interpreted according to the observer. Nor was inclusion body myositis (IBM) identified at the time of Bohan and Peter (1975) criteria proposal.

Diagnostic criteria

There are no universally accepted diagnostic criteria for IIM, although the classification criteria proposed by Bohan and Peter that were originally developed as classification criteria have been widely used in the clinic with the limitations described previously (Bohan and Peter 1975; Box 2.1). Others have been proposed, such as the criteria by Dalakas (1991) and Dalakas and Hohlfeld (2003), and with a greater focus on muscle biopsy features.

Classification criteria

Various classification criteria for IIM have been published. The first data-derived multicentre and multispecialty classification criteria were the Tanimoto criteria for PM and DM (Tanimoto et al. 1995). They include nine criteria items:

- rashes (heliotrope rash or Gottron's sign or linear extensor erythema);
- proximal muscle weakness;
- elevated serum levels of creatine kinase or aldolase;
- muscle pain on grasping or spontaneous muscle pain;
- myogenic changes on electromyography (EMG);
- anti-Jo-1 autoantibody positivity;
- non-destructive arthritis or arthralgia;
- systemic inflammatory signs;
- muscle biopsy evidence of myositis.

These criteria did not include IBM, juvenile myositis, or cancer-associated myositis.

Targoff and colleagues (Targoff et al. 1997) proposed a modification of the Bohan and Peter criteria by including all known myositis-specific antibodies, in addition to magnetic resonance imaging of muscle and a definition of the skin rashes—heliotrope rash or Gottron's sign, or Gottron's papules. Distinction between PM and DM was made by the absence or presence of any of the rashes. Juvenile IIM was defined as age of onset of symptoms <18 years, and IBM was defined as fulfilling the Griggs criteria (Griggs et al. 1995).

In 2004 experts within the European Neuromuscular Centre (ENMC) and Muscle Study Group (MSG) took a new approach, and proposed classification criteria for IIM with detailed description on both inclusion and exclusion features (Hoogendijk et al. 2004). Magnetic resonance imaging of muscle, type, and age of disease onset, presence of myositis-specific antibodies, EMG analyses, and muscle biopsy features revealed by electron microscopy were added to conventional features, including muscle weakness, skin rash, and muscle biopsy findings. These criteria enabled classification of amyopathic DM, non-specific myositis, and necrotizing autoimmune myopathy, in addition to PM and DM.

Although several important attempts to establish diagnostic or classification criteria for IIM have been made, there are currently no universally accepted or properly validated criteria. This was the aim of a large international and multidisciplinary collaboration, which will be discussed later.

IBM from histopathological to clinically based criteria

IBM is classified together with PM and DM as an IIM, although there are distinct clinical features that distinguish IBM from PM and DM, particularly early involvement of asymmetric finger flexor and knee extensor weakness, and resistance to immunosuppressive treatment. The clinical features at presentation and during disease course in patients with IBM are more sensitive than the histopathological features in establishing diagnosis (Brady et al. 2013). This is discussed in more detail in Chapter 11.

It has been debated whether IBM is a primary autoimmune disease or a primary degenerative myopathy, where the lack of demonstrated autoantibodies in IBM patients has favoured a degenerative condition. In 2011, a novel autoantibody directed against a muscle protein, highly specific for IBM patients was found (Salajegheh et al. 2011). The target autoantigen was identified as cytosolic 5'-nucleotidase (cN1A; Larman et al. 2013; Pluk et al. 2013). Autoantibodies against cN1A represent a promising biomarker for IBM that could have significant utility in clinical practice.

Development of new classification criteria for IIM— a case-based procedure

The international myositis interest group, International Myositis Assessment and Clinical Studies (IMACS) group was established in 1999 to facilitate myositis research through international collaboration, such as the development and validation of new outcome measures for use in clinical trials (Rider et al. 2004). Through the IMACS network, an international and multidisciplinary collaboration was initiated in 2004 in order to develop and validate new classification criteria. The multidisciplinary collaboration, the International Myositis Classification Criteria Project (IMCCP), was established with the aim to develop joint classification criteria for adult and juvenile onset IIM that would distinguish them from other mimicking conditions, as well as separating the major IIM subgroups from each other (Lundberg et al. 2016). A steering committee consisting of rheumatologists, paediatric rheumatologists, dermatologists, neurologists, epidemiologists, and biostatisticians was established, which defined the potential criterions, and data to be collected, based on previously published myositis criteria and expert opinion through the network of the IMACS group. Inclusion criteria for IIM cases and comparators in the study were, in order of priority:

- Patient diagnosed for at least 6 months.
- Physician certain of diagnosis—either known IIM or, as comparators, known non-IIM cases, where myositis was considered in the initial differential diagnosis.
- Patients with the most recent and complete data chosen first.

The project involved 47 clinics worldwide (23 from Europe, 17 from North America, one from South America, and six from Asia). Data on clinical, laboratory, and muscle biopsy features from 976 IIM patients (74.5% adults, 25.5% juveniles) and 624 comparators (81.6% adults, 18.4% juveniles) were collected in a database. Data were retrieved from patients with juvenile DM ($n = 248$) and adult PM (n = 245), DM (n = 239), IBM (n = 176), amyopathic DM (n = 44), hypomyopathic DM (n = 12), necrotizing autoimmune myopathy (n = 11), and juvenile PM (n = 1), as well as from patients with a broad spectrum of comparator muscle conditions. Initially, the crude association with IIM for each data variable was assessed. Variables demonstrating high association with IIM and with reasonably high observation frequency (>half of sample size) were selected for further analysis. The reason for this was that classification criteria should preferentially consist of variables that are feasible and routinely used in clinical practice, and should not impose extra burden or expenses for a caregiver or patient. Three techniques were explored for derivation of classification criteria:

- Sum-of-items model in which a patient is classified as being a case if he/ she has a specified number of items from a set of items, similar to the Bohan and Peter criteria.
- Classification tree.
- Probability-score model.

The ensuing candidate criteria were scrutinized with respect to clinical relevance and statistical performance throughout the process. Sixteen variables that in combination and using the probability-score model had the optimal capacity to distinguish IIM from non-IIM cases were identified (Box 2.2). These variables demonstrated different predictive capacities and were therefore given different scores in the final classification criteria.

Box 2.2 The EULAR/ACR classification criteria for adult and juvenile idiopathic inflammatory myopathies

When no better explanation for the symptoms and signs exists these classification criteria can be used

Variable	Score Points		Definition
	Without muscle biopsy	With muscle biopsy	
Age of onset			
Age of onset of first symptom assumed to be related to the disease ≥ 18 years and < 40 years	1.3	1.5	18 ≤ Age (years) at onset of first symptom assumed to be related to the disease < 40
Age of onset of first symptom assumed to be related to the disease ≥ 40 years	2.1	2.2	Age (years) at onset of first symptom assumed to be related to the disease ≥ 40

continued >

Muscle weakness			
Objective symmetric weakness, usually progressive, of the proximal upper extremities	0.7	0.7	Weakness of proximal upper extremities as defined by manual muscle testing or other objective strength testing, which is present on both sides and is usually progressive over time
Objective symmetric weakness, usually progressive, of the proximal lower extremities	0.8	0.5	Weakness of proximal lower extremities as defined by manual muscle testing or other objective strength testing, which is present on both sides and is usually progressive over time
Neck flexors are relatively weaker than neck extensors	1.9	1.6	Muscle grades for neck flexors are relatively lower than neck extensors as defined by manual muscle testing or other objective strength testing
In the legs proximal muscles are relatively weaker than distal muscles	0.9	1.2	Muscle grades for proximal muscles in the legs are relatively lower than distal muscles in the legs as defined by manual muscle testing or other objective strength testing
Skin manifestations			
Heliotrope rash	3.1	3.2	Purple, lilac-colored or erythematous patches over the eyelids or in a periorbital distribution, often associated with periorbital edema
Gottron´s papules	2.1	2.7	Erythematous to violaceous papules over the extensor surfaces of joints, which are sometimes scaly. May occur over the finger joints, elbows, knees, malleoli and toes
Gottron's sign	3.3	3.7	Erythematous to violaceous macules over the extensor surfaces of joints, which are not palpable

Box 2.2 The EULAR/ACR classification criteria for adult and juvenile idiopathic inflammatory myopathies   (continued)

Other clinical manifestations			
Dysphagia or esophageal dysmotility	0.7	0.6	Difficulty in swallowing or objective evidence of abnormal motility of the esophagus
Laboratory measurements			
Anti-Jo-1 (anti-histidyl-tRNA synthetase) autoantibody present	3.9	3.8	Autoantibody test in serum performed with standardized and validated test, showing positive result
Elevated serum levels of creatine kinase (CK)* or lactate dehydrogenase (LDH)* or aspartate aminotransferase (ASAT/AST/SGOT)* or alanine aminotransferase (ALAT/ALT/SGPT)*	1.3	1.4	The most abnormal test values during the disease course (highest absolute level of enzyme) above the relevant upper limit of normal
Muscle biopsy features- presence of:			
Endomysial infiltration of mononuclear cells surrounding, but not invading, myofibres		1.7	Muscle biopsy reveals endomysial mononuclear cells abutting the sarcolemma of otherwise healthy, non-necrotic muscle fibers, but there is no clear invasion of the muscle fibers
Perimysial and/or perivascular infiltration of mononuclear cells		1.2	Mononuclear cells are located in the perimysium and/or located around blood vessels (in either perimysial or endomysial vessels)
Perifascicular atrophy		1.9	Muscle biopsy reveals several rows of muscle fibers which are smaller in the perifascicular region than fibers more centrally located
Rimmed vacuoles		3.1	Rimmed vacuoles are bluish by Hematoxylin and Eosin staining and reddish by modified Gomori-Trichrome stains

*Serum levels above the upper limit of normal.

The summed score from the features present in a patient can be converted into a probability of having IIM using an online web-calculator (www.imm.ki.se/bio-statistics/calculators/iim). In order to avoid unwarranted muscle biopsies, in particular in the context of juvenile patients with typical DM skin manifestations, two sets of classification criteria were developed, one with and one without muscle biopsy features. As recommended by the IMCCP steering committee, when no typical DM skin manifestations (heliotrope rash, Gottron's papules, or Gottron's sign) are evident, muscle biopsy features should be included in the classification of a patient. The best statistical performance was obtained for a 55% probability cut-off for both sets of criteria, thus this cut-off is recommended by the IMCCP steering committee for classification of IIM. As clinical trials require particularly homogeneous patient populations with high specificity, a cut-off of ≥90%, defined as *definite* IIM, was issued by the IMCCP steering committee. Probabilities ranging from ≥55% to <90% were defined as *probable* IIM, whereas probabilities ranging from ≥50% to <55% were defined as *possible* IIM.

The new criteria provide investigators with flexibility in the number of variables to assess since, once a sufficient probability is reached, there is no obligation to assess potentially remaining variables. After classifying a patient as IIM, a classification tree was developed that separates the IIM subclasses DM, amyopathic DM, juvenile DM, PM, and IBM. It should be noted that too few patients with necrotizing autoimmune myopathy were included in the study; therefore, this group of patients is currently part of the PM subgroup in the classification tree. Similarly, identification of juvenile IIM, other than juvenile DM, was not possible due to the limited number of patients available for testing in this subgroup.

The new classification criteria for IIM were compared with previous myositis criteria in the context of statistical performance and showed superior characteristics, with the exception of the Targoff classification criteria (Targoff et al. 1997) that also demonstrated excellent performance. However, the Targoff criteria are based on assessment on more variables, including muscle biopsy and EMG, as well as the obligation of assessing all included variables, making them less flexible. In addition, the subgroup of amyopathic DM was not included in the Targoff criteria, nor are the included variables defined leading to ad hoc interpretations. Finally, these criteria are based on expert opinion and not derived from data on real patients.

SUGGESTED FURTHER READING

Aggarwal R, Ringold S, Khanna D, et al. (2015). Distinctions between diagnostic and classification criteria? *Arthritis Care Res*; **67**: 891–7.

Betteridge Z, McHugh N. (2016). Myositis-specific autoantibodies: an important tool to support diagnosis of myositis. *J Intern Med*; **280**: 8–23.

REFERENCES

Bohan A, Peter JB (1975). Polymyositis and dermatomyositis (parts 1 and 2) (1975). *N Engl J Med*; **292**: 344–7, 403–7.

Brady S, Squier W, Hilton-Jones D (2013). Clinical assessment determines the diagnosis of inclusion body myositis independently of pathological features. *J Neurol Neurosurg Psychiatry*; **84**: 1240–6.

Dalakas MC (1991). Polymyositis, dermatomyositis and inclusion-body myositis. *N Engl J Med*; **325**: 1487–98.

Dalakas M, Hohlfeld R (2003). Polymyositis and dermatomyositis. *Lancet*; **362**: 971–982.

Griggs RC, Askanas V, DiMauro S, et al. (1995). Inclusion body myositis and myopathies. *Ann Neurol*; **38**: 705–13.

Hoogendijk JE, Amato AA, Lecky BR, et al. (2004). 119th ENMC international workshop: trial design in adult idiopathic inflammatory myopathies, with the exception of inclusion body myositis, 10–12 October 2003, Naarden, The Netherlands. *Neuromuscul Disord*; **14**: 337–45.

Larman BH, Salajegheh M, Nazareno R, et al. (2013). Cytosolic 5'-nucelotidase 1A autoimmunity in sporadic inclusion body myositis. *Ann Neurol*; **73**: 408–18.

Lundberg IE, Miller FW, Tjärnlund A, et al. (2016). Diagnosis and classification of idiopathic inflammatory myopathies. *J Intern Med*; **280**: 39–51.

Pluk H, van Hoeve BJ, van Dooren SH (2013). Autoantibodies to cytosolic 5'-nucleotidase 1A in inclusion body myositis. *Ann Neurol*; **73**: 397–407.

Rider LG, Giannini EH, Brunner HI, et al. (2004). International Myositis Assessment and Clinical Studies Group. International consensus on preliminary definitions of improvement in adult and juvenile myositis. *Arthritis Rheum*; **50**: 2281–90.

Salajegheh M, Lam T, Greenberg SA (2011). Autoantibodies against a 43 kDa muscle protein in inclusion body myositis. *PLoS One*; **6**: e20266.

Tanimoto K, Nakano K, Kano S, et al. (1995). Classification criteria for polymyositis and dermatomyositis. *J Rheumatol*; **22**: 668–74.

Targoff IN, Miller FW, Medsger TA, et al. (1997). Classification criteria for the idiopathic inflammatory myopathies. *Curr Opin Rheumatol*; **9**: 527–35.

CHAPTER 3

Aetiology and pathogenesis

Joanna E. Parkes, Simon Rothwell, and Janine A. Lamb

KEY POINTS

- The aetiology and pathogenesis of idiopathic inflammatory myopathies (IIM) is poorly understood; IIM are thought to result from exposure to environmental factors in genetically susceptible individuals.
- Both innate and adaptive immune responses, such as pro-inflammatory cytokines and development of autoantibodies, are involved in IIM.
- There is increasing evidence that non-inflammatory mechanisms including endoplasmic reticulum stress, reactive oxygen species, hypoxia, and impaired autophagy play an important role in IIM pathology.
- Several environmental risk factors, such as infectious agents, ultraviolet radiation, cigarette smoking, and exposure to statins, have been associated with IIM.
- The strongest genetic associations in IIM are within the major histocompatibility complex (MHC), in particular with genes of the 8.1 ancestral haplotype.
- Recent large scale genome wide scans have identified non-MHC associations that overlap with other seropositive autoimmune diseases, commonly implicating genes that regulate the adaptive immune response.
- Integrating data from immunological, genetic, non-inflammatory, and environmental models in IIM will lead to refined models of disease pathogenesis, necessary for improved diagnosis, and to identify patient subgroups for stratified treatment.

Introduction

Disease pathogenesis in idiopathic inflammatory myopathies (IIM) is poorly understood, and the cause is unknown in the large majority of patients. IIM have a complex aetiology, likely resulting from the interplay of environmental risk factors in genetically susceptible individuals. Different disease mechanisms may predominate in the different clinical subgroups. Improved understanding of the pathogenesis of IIM is necessary to gain mechanistic insights and to enable the development of more targeted therapeutic treatments.

Innate and adaptive immunity in IIM

The immune system plays an essential role in host defence against harmful antigens, and in the balance between tolerance and immunity to antigens. Autoimmune disorders arise due to destruction of normal tissue by the immune system, due to failure of the immune system to discriminate between self and non-self-antigens (self-tolerance), leading to an excessive or inappropriate immune response. Both innate and adaptive immune mechanisms are thought to be central to the pathogenesis of autoimmune disorders, including IIM, through highly integrated and interdependent mechanisms.

The innate immune system

The innate immune system is the first line of defence against pathogens, through an immediate non-specific response to foreign bacterial and viral infectious agents, such as phagocytosis or endocytosis by macrophages and neutrophils. A highly conserved set of pattern-recognition receptors, such as Toll-like receptors (TLR), recognize pathogen-associated molecular patterns (PAMPs) on exogenous microorganisms, or endogenous damage associated molecular patterns (DAMPs) released during tissue injury and necrosis, prompting a defensive response by the cell (Figure 3.1). TLRs initiate the inflammatory response primarily through activation of the nuclear factor-kB (NF-kB) pathway, which regulates pro-inflammatory genes and leads to inhibition of muscle regeneration. Inflammatory cytokines, such as interleukin 1 or tumour necrosis factor, released from cells via the innate and adaptive immune systems, and from regenerating myocytes within myositis muscle, play a role in IIM pathogenesis. Chemokines such as chemokine (C-C motif) ligand 2 (CCL2) also may have a role in IIM and regulate the immune response through recruitment of effector immune cells to sites of inflammation. The activity of plasmacytoid dendritic cells (pDCs) is increased in patients with IIM; pDCs are involved in recognition of pathogens and intracellular processing by autophagy, and also produce Type 1 interferons, which mediate the early innate immune response to viral infections. Interferon pathways are strongly upregulated in patients with IIM, particularly in dermatomyositis (DM), and a correlation between serum and muscle IFNα levels, and disease activity has been demonstrated. Innate immunity therefore provides a link to environmental triggers of disease and may identify targets for disease prevention.

The adaptive immune system

In contrast to the innate immune system, the adaptive immune system is initiated by highly specific receptors, selected for reactivity to millions of distinct foreign antigens, and by the formation of immunologic memory to prior exposures. The large and diverse set of recognition molecules includes T-cell receptors and antibodies produced by B-cells. Many autoimmune disorders seem to result from a failure of T-cell tolerance, leading to uncontrolled self-reactivity. As shown in Figure 3.1, a role for T-cells has been identified in IIM, through infiltration of T-cells into affected muscle tissue, which may lead to cytokine production and cytotoxicity to the surrounding muscle fibres. Activation of CD4+ T-cells results in differentiation into different T-helper cell subsets. Th1 cells are produced in

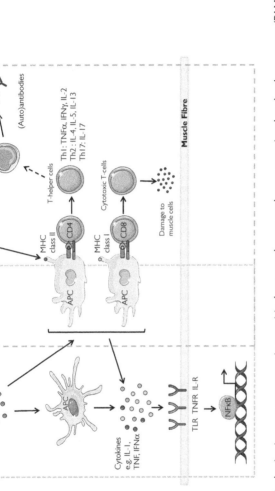

Figure 3.1 The innate and adaptive immune responses in myositis. *Innate:* pathogen or damage associated molecular patterns (PAMPs/DAMPs) are recognized by receptors such as Toll-like receptors (TLRs) on antigen presenting cells (APCs). As a result these cells release cytokines such as interleukin 1 (IL-1), tumour necrosis factor (TNF) or interferon alpha (IFNα) which are recognized by receptors on muscle fibres. TLRs activate the nuclear factor-κB (NF-κB) pathway, which regulates pro-inflammatory genes and leads to inhibition of muscle regeneration. *Adaptive:* antigen presenting cells (APCs) activate CD4+ T-cells via MHC class II and CD8+ T-cells via MHC class I presentation and co-stimulation. Activated CD4+ T-cells can differentiate into different T-helper cell subsets which produce different cytokines. Th2 cells can stimulate B cells into becoming plasma cells that produce antibodies. Activated CD8+ T-cells differentiate into cytotoxic T-cells and damage the muscle fibre via release of perforin-1 and granzyme-B enzymes.

the presence of IL-12 and are associated with IFNγ production. Th2 cells are produced in the presence of IL-4, generate further IL-4 and other cytokines, including IL-5 and IL-13, and stimulate the differentiation of B-cells into antibody-producing plasma cells. Th17 cells are produced in the presence of TGF-β and release cytokines including IL-17.

The role of molecules involved in B-cell activation may reflect a primary pathogenic role of autoantibodies in IIM, although it is not yet clear whether antibodies are a cause or consequence of disease. In IIM, >20 circulating myositis-specific and myositis-associated autoantibodies have been identified, directed against cytoplasmic or nuclear components involved in key intracellular regulatory processes, such as protein synthesis, translation, and chromatin remodelling. These autoantibodies are associated with specific clinical phenotypes, and represent remarkably accurate biomarkers of disease progression and response to treatment. For example, antibodies against IFIH1 (interferon induced with helicase C domain, also known as MDA5) are associated with a rapidly progressive interstitial lung disease with clinically amyopathic dermatomyositis in adult Japanese patients. IFIH1, an intracellular pattern recognition receptor for viral double stranded RNA, is involved in the IFNα pathway, again providing a link between a role of both the innate and adaptive immune systems in IIM.

Non-inflammatory mechanisms in idiopathic inflammatory myopathies

The severity of muscle weakness does not always correlate with inflammation in IIM patients and muscle weakness may persist in patients who have had successful treatment for inflammation. This has led to suggestions that non-inflammatory mechanisms are also involved in IIM such as endoplasmic reticulum (ER) stress, reactive oxygen species, hypoxia, and impaired autophagy.

ER stress occurs when there is build-up of unprocessed or misfolded proteins in the ER lumen. An indicator of ER stress, Glucose related protein 78 (GRP78), has been detected on the cell surface, in the cytoplasm, and is widely spread over the sarcolemma and sarcoplasm of muscle fibres in polymyositis (PM) and DM patients. ER stress in IIM may be induced by overexpression of major histocompatibility complex (MHC) Class I, which occurs in 75% of IIM patients, on the cell surface and sarcoplasmic reticulum of skeletal muscle cells. ER stress activates NF-κB, which in turn upregulates target genes including endogenous MHC Class I, forming a positive feedback loop as MHC Class I further induces ER stress. NF-κB inhibits the myogenic regulatory factor MyoD, thereby reducing myoblast differentiation, and promotes expression of pro-inflammatory cytokines causing damage to muscle fibres. Induction of ER stress by overexpression of MHC Class I is used in the H-2k^b mouse model of myositis and results in muscle weakness, damage, and inflammation often accompanied by autoantibodies.

Reactive oxygen species (ROS) are generated during protein folding and are normally regulated by antioxidants. However, the increase in folding attempts under ER stress results in overwhelming levels of ROS, which can then leave the ER and cause oxidative damage to contractile and other proteins. ER stress can also induce increased calcium transport to the mitochondria where increased respiration also generates ROS.

Hypoxia also is implicated in IIM by observation of reduced capillary density and expression of a hypoxia marker, high mobility group protein B1 (HMGB1), in muscle fibres of IIM patients in the absence of inflammation. Hypoxia has been found to alter ROS generation and can lead to increased levels of hydrogen peroxide in skeletal muscle, which may contribute to muscle damage. Furthermore, overexpression of vascular endothelial growth factor, erythropoietin, hypoxia inducible factor 1α, and their respective receptors have been detected in muscle from IIM patients. Hypoxia is linked to muscle weakness due to the resultant reduction in ATP and phosphocreatine.

Normally, proteins are removed from cells by autophagy if not required or damaged. Autophagosomes transport these proteins to lysosomes for degradation. Failure of this pathway may result in cell death. Accumulation of microtubule-associated protein 1A/1B-light chain 3 (LC3), a marker of autophagy, has been reported in muscle of PM patients with mitochondrial pathology and in inclusion body myositis (IBM) patients. This may indicate that LC3 is overexpressed as a result of increased or incorrect autophagy. Impaired autophagy could explain some of the characteristics of IIM including accumulation of mitochondria with mutated DNA, protein aggregates seen in IBM, and altered antigen presentation in the form of MHC Class I on muscle fibres.

The role of environmental risk factors in IIM

The role of infectious agents in IIM

The mechanisms for development of autoimmunity following infection are unclear and it is not yet established whether infection is primary or secondary to the immune changes. The spectrum of infectious agents reported includes microbial pathogens, such as viruses, bacteria, fungi, and parasites. Epstein-Barr virus is one of the most frequently reported viruses implicated in the development of IIM, together with other autoimmune diseases. Other viruses reported include retroviruses, such as HIV, hepatitis, and influenza viruses and enteroviruses, such as coxsackie viruses. Viral involvement is supported by the upregulated interferon pathways observed in IIM (see Innate and Adaptive Immunity in IIM). Bacteria reported to be associated with IIM include *Mycobacterium tuberculosis*, *Staphylococcus aureus*, and streptococcal infection. Further evidence for the potential role of infectious agents in IIM comes from their use in the development of experimental animal models of myositis.

Increasingly, the role of the host microenvironment in development of auto-immunity is being investigated through studies of the microbiome; the combined genetic material of the microorganisms in a particular environment, for example, in the human gut or on the skin.

The role of non-infectious environmental factors in idiopathic inflammatory myopathies

There have been reports of spatial clustering, the role of ultraviolet radiation with a latitudinal gradient of increasing prevalence from north to south reported in DM, and of the DM specific antibody anti-Mi-2. Seasonal onset has been reported in juvenile dermatomyositis (JDM). The frequency of the most common adult myositis-specific autoantibody, anti-Jo-1, is increased in cigarette smoking individuals who are positive for the *HLA-DRB1*03* allele, suggesting a risk-inducing gene-environment interaction similar to that seen in rheumatoid arthritis. Similarly, *HLA-DRB1*11* positive individuals have an increased risk of developing anti-HMGCR antibody positive immune-mediated necrotizing myopathy as a result of exposure to statins. The reason for the association between myositis and cancer is still unknown; the increased risk of cancer observed in IIM, with paraneoplastic myopathy occurring as a result of the malignancy, may be due to environmental factors that act as both carcinogens and inflammatory triggers. It has been suggested that autoantigen mutation in the patient's cancer triggers an autoimmune anti-tumour cytolytic response, which in some patients successfully eliminates the cancer.

Genetic risk factors in idiopathic inflammatory myopathies

Initial evidence for genetic susceptibility to IIM comes from the observation that there is an increased risk of autoimmune disease in first degree relatives of those with IIM and rare case reports of familial aggregation. To investigate genes involved in disease, genetic association studies are used to compare the frequency of genetic variants between disease and healthy populations.

The role of major histocompatibility complex genes in idiopathic inflammatory myopathies

To date, the strongest genetic associations found in IIM are within the MHC, in particular within MHC class I and class II genes that code for proteins that present antigens to the immune system to trigger an immune response. Genes within the MHC are highly variable across the population and are inherited in gene blocks called haplotypes. The strongest association is with the 8.1 ancestral haplotype, a common haplotype in Caucasian populations that has been found to confer susceptibility to many autoimmune diseases. Recent studies suggest that multiple alleles on this haplotype may independently contribute to IIM risk, in particular

*HLA-DRB1*03:01* and *HLA-B*08:01*. There is also evidence that risk within these alleles may be explained by certain amino-acid positions that affect the structure of the peptide binding pocket, affecting the ability to bind antigenic peptides, and present them to the T-cell receptor. Unique MHC associations have been found with myositis specific autoantibodies, supported by the observation that myositis specific antibodies are almost mutually exclusive. In this way, it seems that genotype may predict serotype, which in turn may predict phenotype.

The role of non-major histocompatibility complex genes in idiopathic inflammatory myopathies

As many autoimmune diseases share common associations within the MHC, it is hypothesized that other genes independent of this region will contribute to specific disease susceptibility. Early candidate genes studies in IIM were typically small, and focused on genes known to be associated with other autoimmune diseases and/or those with biological rationale. An emphasis on coordinated case ascertainment has facilitated larger and more meaningful genetic studies. A genome-wide association study in DM and a follow-up targeted fine-mapping study in PM and DM confirms that there is extensive genetic overlap between IIM and other autoimmune diseases. Reassuringly, many of these associations have been replicated in other ethnic populations, such as Chinese and Japanese, suggesting a common aetiology.

PM and DM share genetic risk factors involved in the adaptive immune response, such as *STAT4* and *UBE2L3* that are known regulators of T and B cell differentiation respectively. However, specific genetic associations, such as the *PTPN22* gene in PM, which is involved in T cell signalling, and *BLK* in DM, which is involved in B-cell activation, suggest a different genetic architecture underpinning these subgroups of IIM. Candidate gene studies in IBM have focused on genes associated with neurodegenerative diseases such as Alzheimer's disease, and genes previously implicated in the Mendelian forms of IBM known as hereditary IBM. However, these have failed to find significant associations.

For most genetic associations in IIM, how these variants contribute to disease pathogenesis is currently unknown. For some genes, such as *PTPN22*, the variant may directly affect gene function. For others, genetic variants may have an indirect effect, for example altering expression of genes that result in dysregulation of key immune pathways, leading to a break in tolerance of the immune system and a subsequent autoimmune phenotype.

Translational relevance

In summary, the aetiology and pathogenesis of IIM currently is poorly understood, and different disease mechanisms may predominate in the different IIM subtypes. Both innate and adaptive immune responses, such as pro-inflammatory cytokines and the development of autoantibodies, have been shown to be involved. There is increasing evidence that non-inflammatory mechanisms including endoplasmic reticulum stress, hypoxia, reactive oxygen species, and impaired autophagy play an important role in disease pathology. IIM are thought to result from exposure to environmental factors, such as infectious agents, ultraviolet radiation, cigarette smoking, and exposure to statins. The IIM likely share a similar genetic architecture with other autoimmune diseases; a substantial proportion of the genetic risk lies within the MHC, whilst genes outside of the MHC region have also been implicated.

Integrating data from immunological, genetic, non-inflammatory, and environmental models in IIM will potentially lead to increasingly refined and integrated models of disease pathogenesis. Improved understanding of the aetiology and pathogenesis of IIM is necessary for earlier detection, improved diagnostic accuracy and prediction of disease progression, and to identify clinically meaningful patient subgroups for stratified treatment approaches. Ultimately, this knowledge may implicate new pathways that enable the development of more targeted novel therapeutic agents.

SUGGESTED READING

Ceribelli A, De Santis M, Isailovic N, et al. (2017). The immune response and the pathogenesis of idiopathic inflammatory myositis: a critical review. *Clin Rev Allergy Immunol*; **52**(1): 58–70.

Moran EM, Mastaglia FL. (2014). Cytokines in immune-mediated inflammatory myopathies: cellular sources, multiple actions and therapeutic implications. *Clin Exp Immunol*; **178**: 405–415.

Higgs BW, Liu Z, White B, et al. (2011). Patients with systemic lupus erythematosus, myositis, rheumatoid arthritis and scleroderma share activation of a common type I interferon pathway. *Ann Rheum Dis*; **70**: 2029–36.

Betteridge Z, McHugh N. (2015). Myositis-specific autoantibodies: an important tool to support diagnosis of myositis. (Review Symposium.) *J Intern Med*; **280**: 8–23.

Meyer A, Meyer, N, Schaeffer M, et al. (2015). Incidence and prevalence of inflammatory myopathies: a systematic review. *Rheumatology*; **54**: 50–63.

Lightfoot AP, McArdle A, Jackson MJ, et al. (2015). In the idiopathic inflammatory myopathies (IIM), do reactive oxygen species (ROS) contribute to muscle weakness? *Ann Rheum Dis*; **74**: 1340–6.

Temiz P, Weihl CC, Pestronk A. (2009). Inflammatory myopathies with mitochondrial pathology and protein aggregates. *J Neurol Sci*; **278**: 25–9.

Gan L, Miller FW. (2011). State of the art: what we know about infectious agents and myositis. *Curr Opin Rheumatol*; **23**: 585–94.

Rothwell S, Cooper RG, Lundberg IE, et al. (2015). Dense genotyping of immune-related loci in idiopathic inflammatory myopathies confirms HLA alleles as the strongest genetic risk factor and suggests different genetic background for major clinical subgroups. *Ann Rheum Dis*; **75**: 1558–66.

Kirino Y, Remmers EF. (2015). Genetic architectures of seropositive and seronegative rheumatic diseases. *Nat Rev Rheumatol*; **11**: 401–14.

CHAPTER 3

CHAPTER 4

Extramuscular complications occurring in myositis

Jens Schmidt

KEY POINTS

- Extramuscular organs predominantly affected in myositis are the skin, lungs, joints, and heart.
- Skin features are usually not a serious problem, but their pattern may greatly facilitate accurate identification of subtypes within the myositis spectrum.
- Pulmonary manifestations include interstitial lung disease (ILD) and pulmonary hypertension.
- Involvement of the joints can include a polyarthritis pattern mimicking rheumatoid arthritis.
- Heart involvement in myositis may include conduction defects, serositis, cardiomyositis, cardiomyopathy, and right heart failure.
- Dysphagia in myositis can be severe and associated with choking or aspiration pneumonia. In some cases dysphagia can be the sole presenting symptom of myositis.

Introduction

It is important to point out that idiopathic inflammatory myopathies (IIM) cases with extra-muscular manifestation only rarely are regarded as 'connective tissue disease (CTD)-overlap cases. CTD-overlap is a term used to describe patients in whom features from multiple, defined CTDs overlap in well recognized patterns and associations. For instance, patients with 'mixed connective tissue disease' (MCTD, also known as Sharp's syndrome) exhibit prominent features of scleroderma, interstitial lung disease, and myositis, but where the prominence of any individual CTD will vary between each case. Furthermore, another feature of MCTD is the presence of anti-U1-RNP antibodies. These are relatively specific for MCTD, and their detection would not be expected in pure rheumatoid arthritis, systemic sclerosis, or Sjögren's Syndrome. In general, IIM are more likely to occur as a distinct clinical phenotype rather than in conjunction with another CTD. It has to be acknowledged that the definitions of CTD, overlap syndrome, and IIM with extra-muscular manifestations are not precise and an international consensus is lacking. It is an inherent problem that there is a considerable overlap in the use of these terms.

Skin

Spectrum of changes

Skin changes are common in patients with IIM and can greatly help in securing a subgroup diagnosis within the IIM disease spectrum, often without the need for a skin or muscle biopsy. However, skin changes can also start non-specifically with an undefined pattern and may only become more characteristic over time. In hallmark dermatomyositis (DM), pathognomonic features include a raised, violaceous rash over the dorsum of the finger proximal/distal interphalangeal joints (Gottron's sign), a heliotrope (lilac or violaceous) rash over the upper eyelids and sometimes of the lower eyelids, an erythematous rash on the back and front of the upper chest (shawl and V-signs, respectively), a violaceous or erythematous rash over the extensor surfaces of the elbows and knees, and dermal erothema of other areas of the body, including the cheeks and forehead. Not all of these rashes will always be present, but if Gottron's papules and/or a heliotrope are present, this is thought diagnostic of DM, even in the absence of muscle disease (amyopathic DM; **see** Figs 4.1 and 4.2). In patients with DM or polymyositis (PM), the presence of painful and cracked skin over the radial aspects of the thumb and index fingers (mechanics' hands) may provide clues to an underlying antisynthetase syndrome (ASS; see next section).

Some IIM patients also possess systemic sclerosis (SSc)-related antibodies such as anti-PM-Scl; these cases rarely get mechanics' hands, but they do develop

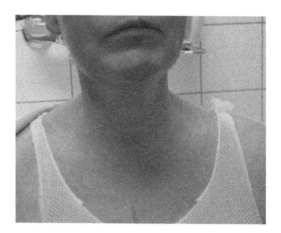

Figure 4.1 Characteristic skin feature in a patient with dermatomyositis: erythematous rash on the face, neck, and anterior chest (V sign). See Colour Plate Section.

Reproduced from de Hilton-Jones D and Turner M, *Oxford Textbook of Neuromuscular Disorders* (2014) with permission from Oxford University Press.

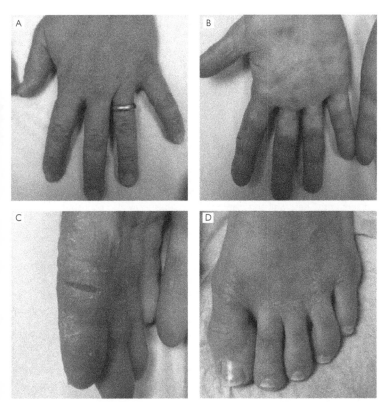

Figure 4.2 Characteristic skin feature in a patient with dermatomyositis: (A) papules on the back of the finger joints (Gottron's sign), (B) palmar erythema, (C) mechanics' hands, and/or (D) mechanics' feet. See Colour Plate Section.

Reproduced from Ciafaloni E et al. (2014). *Evaluation and Treatment of Myopathies* with permission from Oxford University Press.

Raynaud's, ILD, and mild cutaneous SSc, usually limited to the hands and sometimes the forearms.

As with the presence of other comorbidities and organ involvement, the autoantibody status often helps to underpin the diagnosis in the IIM. The importance of serological testing to further facilitate subtype identification of an individual case is detailed below and in Chapter 12, where a key message is that the serological IIM-phenotypes should be regarded as distinct from other defined CTDs, including MCTD.

With the identification of many new antibodies in recent years, it has become clear that certain antibody specificities are associated with a typical pattern of organ involvement, e.g. skin, joint, or lung. Antibodies associated with SSc features include anti-Ku and anti-Pm-Scl, both of which can be associated with ILD. Autoantibodies associated with Sjögren's syndrome include anti-U1/U2/U3nRNP, anti-SS-A (Ro), anti-SS-B (La) and anti-Sm (U-snRNPs) antibodies, but these are all rarely found in isolation within primary IIM cases. Anti-Ro antibodies are often present in association with one of the anti-synthetase antibodies.

Lungs

Clinical presentation

Lung disease can often occur as an extra-muscular manifestation of myositis. Different patterns of lung manifestations include ILD, pulmonary hypertension, and serositis. Chest wall and diaphragm weakness may also contribute to shortness of breath, especially when patients are asked to lie flat, the latter due to 'diaphragmatic splinting'. Symptoms of ILD include dyspnoea initially during exercise, but eventually even at rest, troublesome dry and non-productive cough, digital clubbing in some cases, and with asthenia as a late feature of the terminal phase.

A well-recognized clinical presentation is the ASS, which includes any combination of painful and cracked skin over the radial aspects of the thumb and index fingers (mechanics' hands), Raynaud's phenomenon, ILD, low grade inflammatory arthritis, and fever. ASS is associated with the presence of one of the large family of anti-synthetase antibodies, i.e. anti-Jo-1, -PL-7, -PL-12, -Zo, -OJ, -KS, -EJ, and -Ha. Lung involvement may also be observed in patients possessing anti-PmScl and anti-MDA5 antibodies (see Chapter 12). MDA-5 antibodies are specific for a usually amyopathic DM with deeply ulcerating skin lesions, and an aggressive and rapidly progressive ILD.

The responsiveness of ILD to immunosuppressive therapy varies between individuals, and between ILD subsets. In general terms, CTD-ILD, such as that occurring in the IIM, responds better than rheumatoid arthritis (RA)-ILD or some idiopathic forms.

Diagnostic approach

If symptoms of lung disease or myositis disease-specific antibodies are present and associated with ILD, the patient should undergo pulmonary function tests to determine the total lung capacity, as well as the ventilation and diffusion capacities. The diffusion capacity of the lung for carbon monoxide is typically reduced in ILD, even early on, without deficits in other ventilation assessment parameters. A typical finding in ILD includes a reduced or normal forced expiratory volume in 1 second (FEV_1), an increased FEV_1/FVC (forced vital capacity) ratio, and a reduced TLCO (**transfer** factor for carbon monoxide). However, pulmonary function tests may be difficult to interpret, since lung function may be impaired by different pathomechanisms, including respiratory muscle weakness and pulmonary arterial hypertension. For these reasons, if ILD does complicate an IIM case, the patient should be referred for specialist pulmonary assessment, investigation, and treatment.

A useful diagnostic tool for assessing CTD-ILD is high-resolution computed tomography (HRCT) of the chest, which can typically demonstrate changes in the lower lobes including linear and ground-glass opacity, reticulation, peribronchovascular thickening, areas of small cystic spaces with thickened walls (honeycombing) as well as traction bronchiectasis (Fig. 4.3). However, the assessment

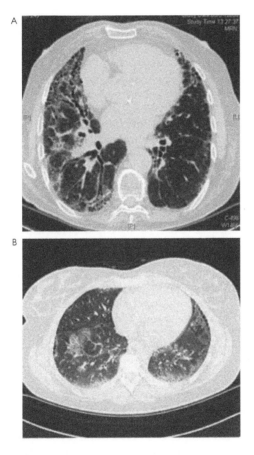

Figure 4.3 High-resolution computed tomography (HRCT) of the chest with different patterns of of an interstitial lung disease (ILD): (A) pulmonary fibrosis (usual interstitial pneumonia, UIP) in a patient with SLE-related ILD; (B) non-specific interstitial pneumonia (NSIP) in a patient with SSc-related ILD.

Reproduced from Watts et al. *Oxford Desk Reference: Rheumatology* (2009) with permission from Oxford University Press.

of HRCT is difficult and should be reserved for those with specialist pulmonary radiological expertise.

Joints: clinical spectrum and diagnostic approach

Arthropathy can particularly present in association with CTD/overlap disease with skin involvement, especially in the ASS. Arthritis symptoms include pain, swelling, and stiffness of joints, and patients develop a chronic reduction of joint movements. Apart from typical involvement of small hand joints, other involved joints include the knee, ankle, wrist, and hips, and it is well recognized that patients initially diagnosed as seronegative RA can eventually be re-diagnosed as ASS when weakness and/or ILD become clinically obvious. Where clinical suspicion of ASS arises in such a patient, diagnostics may include serology testing for anti-nuclear antibody, extractible nuclear antigens, myositis specific antibodies, rheumatoid factor, and anti-citrullinated peptide antibodies. X-ray changes can include joint space narrowing and bone erosions in affected joints to suggest RA, even occasionally in obvious ASS cases.

Oesophagus

Symptoms of dysphagia

In all forms of IIM, i.e. DM, PM, immune-mediated necrotizing myopathy (IMNM), and inclusion body myositis (IBM), the pharyngeal and upper oesophageal muscles can be affected to cause dysphagia. In DM, PM, and IMNM, patients can develop pharyngeal dysphagia subacutely during the onset of their disease; in IBM, the symptoms usually evolve more slowly and usually after years of disease. However, occasionally dysphagia can be the sole presenting symptom in myositis, particularly in IBM. The severity of dysphagia ranges from very mild, with occasional coughing during eating, to a severely impaired passage of food and the requirement for a feeding by tube, or eventually by insertion of a permanent percutaneous endoscopic gastrostomy (PEG) tube. The danger of untreated or unrecognized swallowing impairment is aspiration, which may lead to secondary pneumonia and even death.

Symptoms of dysphagia include repeated clearing of the throat, even unrelated to meals or drinks; coughing during eating; the feeling that 'food gets stuck'; choking; a prolonged duration of the food intake; fear of eating or a change of eating habits, e.g. only small bites or avoid chunks of meat, etc. Attempts to swallow fluids may sometimes be associated with fluid coming down the nose. It is important to note that many patients may not spontaneously report their swallowing symptoms, as some patients do recognize their swallowing behaviour as 'abnormal', but do not associate it as due to their disease. In SSc patients who develop complicating myositis problems, it is important to differentiate pharyngeal weakness from swallowing difficulties arising from lower oesophageal dysmotility, as the investigation and treatment strategies differ considerably between these entities. This distinction can only be made by means of imaging diagnostics (see below).

Diagnostic approach

When symptoms of dysphagia are present, all complaints and severity should be carefully noted for comparison with complaint levels at subsequent visits. If possible, a standardized assessment instrument should be used, such as the Sydney swallowing questionnaire. Diagnostics for dysphagia should include a fibre-optic endoscopic evaluation of swallowing. Affected patients should also undergo videofluoroscopy, a 'functional' X-ray procedure, which radiographically assesses the swallowing of a radiolucent dye (Fig.4.4). This investigation is important to rule out other causes of dysphagia, such as a tumour, or a pharyngeal pouch, stricture or achalasia. Videofluoroscopy can also demonstrate direct causes of the dysphagia, e.g. insufficient opening of the upper oesophageal sphincter in those patients with upper swallowing dysfunction.

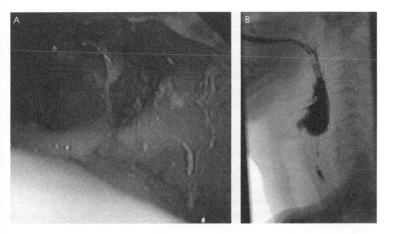

Figure 4.4 Detection of impaired swallowing in a patient with IBM. (A) A grey contrast liquid is visible by fibre-optic endoscopic evaluation of swallowing (FEES) after swallowing. (B) Impaired opening of the upper oesophagus sphincter impairs propulsion of barium liquid in videofluoroscopy,

Heart: spectrum of heart involvement and diagnostic approach

Involvement of the heart is an under-recognized extra-muscular manifestation in the IIM. Two major cardiac problems can occur:

- Cardiomyopathy/cardiomyositis, which are rare, but do occur.
- Conduction defects which can evolve.

Problematic serositis/pericarditis can occur in IIM, but is rare except where more generalized CTD symptoms and signs develop. Increased cardiac mortality is a well-recognized feature of IIM, and relating to issues already discussed, as well as to the increased cardiovascular risks relating to affected patients' chronic inflammation and its treatment. In IBM, cardiomyopathy is thought less common, though this awaits conformation in further studies. Symptoms of heart involvement include: arrhythmias and shortness of breath. The investigation of suspected heart disease should include an electrocardiogram (ECG) and a 24-h ECG to identify conduction blocks and arrhythmias. Echocardiography and, if available, gadolinium-enhanced magnetic resonance imaging, can be used to determine ventricular function, the presence of myocarditis and to identify possible cardiomyopathy. The presence of cardiac involvement should prompt specialist cardiological referral and assessment, and consideration of escalation of immunosuppression.

Treatment

For all extra-muscular complications of myositis, treatment considerations should take into account all organ manifestations and their severity and overall impact on disease outcome. Most extra-muscular complications will respond to an escalating immunosuppressive regimen including:

- Glucocorticoids.
- Azathioprine, methotrexate, or mycophenolate.
- Cyclophosphamide or rituximab especially for treatment of refractory ILD.

Severe dysphagia may require a (temporary) feeding tube through the nose, or a permanent PEG tube to prevent aspiration and so protect against pneumonia. Speech and language therapy, with close assessment and monitoring of swallowing, should be regarded as crucial in patients affected by pharyngeal and oesophageal problems. If symptoms of dysphagia cannot be controlled by the standard systemic immunosuppression, a local therapy such as botulinum toxin injection should be contemplated, but evaluated and delivered by an expert, e.g. by an experienced ear, nose, and throat specialist.

SUGGESTED READING

Betteridge Z, McHugh N (2016). Myositis-specific autoantibodies: an important tool to support diagnosis of myositis. *J Intern Med*; **280**: 8–23.

Clarke JT, Werth VP (2010). Rheumatic manifestations of skin disease. *Curr Opin Rheumatol*; **22**: 78–84.

Hallowell RW, Danoff SK (2014). Interstitial lung disease associated with the idiopathic inflammatory myopathies and the antisynthetase syndrome: recent advances. *Curr Opin Rheumatol*; **26**: 684–9.

Iudici M, van der Goes MC, Valentini G, et al. (2013). Glucocorticoids in systemic sclerosis: weighing the benefits and risks—a systematic review. *Clin Exp Rheumatol*; **31**: 157–65.

Lega JC, Reynaud Q, Belot A, et al. (2015). Idiopathic inflammatory myopathies and the lung. *Eur Respir Rev*; **24**: 216–38.

Magro-Checa C, Zirkzee EJ, Huizinga TW, et al. (2016). Management of neuropsychiatric systemic lupus erythematosus: current approaches and future perspectives. *Drugs*; **76**: 459–83.

Van GH, Charles-Schoeman C. (2014). The heart in inflammatory myopathies. *Rheum Dis Clin North Am*; **40**: 1–10.

Differential diagnosis

CHAPTER 5

Metabolic myopathies

James B. Lilleker and Mark E. Roberts

KEY POINTS

- Metabolic myopathies are rare and can be difficult to diagnose. However, the clinical presentation can be similar to, and thus mimic, both the idiopathic inflammatory myopathies and other genetic muscle disorders such as the muscular dystrophies.

- Careful enquiry about the nature and timing of muscle pain, as well as identification of other clinical 'red-flags', can highlight the possibility of a metabolic myopathy.

- In treatment-resistant 'myositis' or seronegative 'myositis', the possibility of metabolic myopathy or muscular dystrophy mimicking myositis should be considered early.

- Diagnosis of metabolic myopathies depends on a multidisciplinary team, an awareness of the increasing availability of enzyme activity testing and the utility of expanding genetic technologies.

- Dietary manipulation and enzyme replacement therapies are useful treatments in some cases.

Introduction

The metabolic myopathies are a group of genetically determined conditions where defects in the metabolic processes of energy storage and utilization cause exercise intolerance, fatigue, muscle pain, and weakness. Whilst classically presenting in childhood, metabolic myopathies can also present in adulthood, sometimes *de novo*, but also because longstanding symptoms can be dismissed by parents, patients, and physicians. Furthermore, with advancements in molecular genetic diagnostic techniques, late-onset metabolic myopathies are being increasingly recognized, usually with a more restricted phenotype to that classically described. This chapter will focus on metabolic disorders that are more likely to come to the attention of adult physicians, rather than paediatricians.

The metabolic myopathies chiefly comprise the glycogen storage disorders (GSDs), fatty acid oxidation disorders (FAODs), disorders of purine metabolism, and mitochondrial disorders (Box 5.1). Metabolic myopathies are rare, but the true incidence and prevalence are unknown. McArdle disease (GSD type 5) affects around 1 in 100,000 people and Pompe disease (GSD type 2) around 1

Box 5.1 Key metabolic myopathies that can present in adulthood

Glycogen storage disorders (GSD)

- GSD type 2—Pompe disease
- GSD type 3—Debrancher deficiency
- GSD type 5—McArdle disease
- GSD type 7—Tarui disease

Fatty acid oxidation disorders (FAOD)

- Carnitine palmitoyltransferase II (CPTII) deficiency
- Very long chain acyl-CoA dehydrogenase (VLCAD) deficiency

Disorders of purine metabolism

- Myoadenylate Deaminase Deficiency

Mitochondrial disorders

---

in 40,000. The metabolic myopathies represent a significant group of disorders, which can clinically mimic idiopathic inflammatory myopathies (IIM). As specific treatments are now available for certain metabolic myopathies (e.g. Pompe disease), an awareness of key clinical features ('red-flags') to identify them is vital.

When to suspect a metabolic myopathy

A summary of clinical 'red-flags' for metabolic myopathies is outlined in Box 5.2. Due to the transient nature of symptoms in many cases, patients may have no symptoms at the time of review and the serum creatine kinase (CK) level (particularly in those with FAODs) can be normal. Fixed weakness or other abnormal examination findings are also uncommon and therefore the history is of key importance.

The 'right' questions to ask

Exercise intolerance and myalgia

Exercise intolerance due to muscle pain (myalgia) and cramping is a key metabolic symptom. Fasting can also trigger symptoms in the FAODs and mitochondrial disorders. Furthermore, the 'sporting stoic' may have longstanding exercise-induced myalgia, but has assumed that this is a normal phenomenon. Only once an episode of frank rhabdomyolysis has occurred may an individual patient finally seek medical attention. Changes in exercise patterns may also unmask metabolic disorders.

Exercise intolerance is not specific for metabolic myopathies and can be difficult to distinguish from the fatigue of systemic disorders, chronic fatigue syndrome, or fibromyalgia. Fatigue is also very common (but often underappreciated) in IIM and it may also be a feature of the muscular dystrophies, particularly Becker muscular dystrophy (BMD).

Box 5.2 Clinical 'red-flags' for the metabolic myopathies

History

- Episode(s) of rhabdomyolysis
- Episodes(s) of pigmenturia
- Exercise intolerance and fatigue
- Symptoms arising after periods of fasting (e.g. for religious reasons)
- Prominent myalgia, cramps, and stiffness
- Consanguinity

Examination

- Contractures (transient or fixed)
- Ptosis or ophthalmoplegia (mitochondrial disorders)
- Clues to alternative diagnosis (e.g. calf pseudo-hypertrophy seen in Becker muscular dystrophy)

Disease course

- Episodic, exertion related symptoms
- Treatment resistant and/or seronegative 'myositis'

Once a history of exercise-induced myalgia is disclosed, it is important to establish the *type* of activity that produces symptoms. In cases where short bursts of high intensity exertion produce symptoms, GSDs should be considered first. A 'second wind' phenomenon may occur, with a resolution of pain and regaining of muscle strength after resting for around ten minutes, a clue pointing to McArdle disease (GSD type 5). Conversely, symptoms precipitated by prolonged periods of low intensity ('endurance') exercise are more typical of the FAODs.

Rhabdomyolysis

It is important to establish if there have been any episodes of the pigmenturia, which may follow rhabdomyolysis. A misdiagnosis of pigmenturia as a urinary tract infection is possible (presence of urinary myoglobin giving a false positive reading for blood on urine test strips) and there can be a failure to recognize the importance of 'rust'- or 'cola'-coloured urine ("I thought I was just dehydrated"). Additionally, as pigmenturia can be accompanied by fever, vomiting, malaise, and muscle swelling, the cause of rhabdomyolysis can wrongly be attributed to a viral myositis.

Developmental milestones

Clues indicating a genetic myopathy are often found through careful questioning of the patient (and relatives) about distant personal and family history. In adults presenting with a suspected genetic myopathy, symptoms may have been present

for years. There may be recollection of delays in walking ability or poor performance at school sporting events. Exercise-induced myalgia may have been wrongly
labelled as 'growing pains'.

Family history

Simply asking 'does anything run in the family?' may not be adequate. Constructing
a family tree with direct questioning about the possibility of consanguinity is
thus advised and of special importance given that many of the disorders under
consideration here have an autosomal recessive inheritance pattern. Populations
with limited genetic diversity may be at increased risk of recessive genetic diseases, e.g. certain religious groups and populations from isolated geographic
locations. Until recently, many metabolic muscle diseases were not well doc-
umented and many patients would have lived without a diagnosis. Questions
regarding family members should therefore not be limited to diseases *diagnosed*,
but also any suggestive *symptoms,* including exercise intolerance and early use of
walking aids, etc.

Response to previous treatment

Accurately diagnosed IIM cases will at least partly respond to corticosteroid
therapy in most cases. Thus, when an individual case proves truly resistant to
corticosteroids and/or other immunosuppression, particularly in seronegative
'myositis', the diagnosis should be carefully reviewed and consideration given to
the alternative possibility of a genetic myopathy.

Findings on examination

Whilst neurological examination in those with a metabolic myopathy may be
normal, particularly between episodes of symptoms, a thorough examination is
essential as subtle diagnostic clues can sometimes be identified:

Fixed weakness

Permanent weakness, present between bouts of symptoms, can occur in those
with McArdle disease (GSD type 5), where proximal weakness in older patients
may be found, and in Pompe disease (GSD type 2), where weakness can involve
axial musculature (particularly paraspinous) and proximal leg muscles. Scapular
winging and respiratory muscle weakness can also be seen in Pompe disease. The
FAODs less commonly cause fixed weakness.

   Other genetic myopathies mimicking a metabolic myopathy may be associated
with fixed weakness, e.g. mild forms of BMD can present with calf pain on exertion, and proximal arm and leg weakness. The presence of calf hypertrophy, a
reflection of muscle being replaced by fat and connective tissue, is a feature of
BMD, which can be identified on careful evaluation. Myotonic dystrophy type
2 (proximal myotonic myopathy [PROMM]) can also mimic a metabolic myopathy, often presenting with exercise-induced myalgia and cramping. Proximal limb

weakness, and sometimes facial muscle weakness, cataracts, deafness, and heart rhythm abnormalities are other clues to a diagnosis of PROMM.

Contractures

Contractures are shortening of muscles that restrict movement about a joint. In metabolic myopathies, contractures are usually transient and painful, in contrast to painless, fixed contractures in the muscular dystrophies. Painful transient contractures classically occur in McArdle disease (GSD type 5), usually in the context of high intensity anaerobic exercise. The induced energy deficit means that normal muscle relaxation, also an energy dependent process, cannot optimally occur. Muscle ischaemia resulting from prolonged and intense contractions causes muscle pain and damage, which may be severe. However, fixed contractures can occur in the metabolic myopathies, particularly Pompe disease (GSD type 2), and also after an episode of rhabdomyolysis from any cause. Fixed contractures might also be a clue to genetic muscular dystrophy mimicking metabolic myopathy. For example, BMD and limb girdle muscular dystrophy type 2I (LGMD2I—FKRP myopathy) are associated with contractures, and can present with muscle pain and rhabdomyolysis.

Ptosis and ophthalmoplegia

In this context, identification of ptosis and ophthalmoplegia, often subtle (e.g. perhaps only recognized when examining old photographs), may point towards a diagnosis of a mitochondrial disease. In addition to exercise intolerance, mitochondrial diseases are often associated with hearing loss, epilepsy, cognitive impairment, neuropathy, or retinopathy.

Multisystem disease

Cardiac involvement is common in early-onset Pompe disease (GSD type 2), but less so in late-onset form. Otherwise, cardiac disease is generally not seen in either the GSDs or FAODs. The presence of heart involvement may also be a clue to a metabolic myopathy mimic, such as BMD. Respiratory muscle weakness is a common feature of late-onset Pompe disease and may present insidiously with nocturnal hypoventilation. Cerebral artery aneurysms can also be seen and presentation with subarachnoid haemorrhage can be the prompt to eventually diagnosing Pompe disease. Co-existing epilepsy, migraine, stroke-like episodes, hearing loss, and/or diabetes may provide clues to underlying mitochondrial disease.

Investigations

Early involvement of an experienced multidisciplinary team comprising neuromuscular specialists, including neurologists and rheumatologists, as well as neurophysiologists, metabolic medicine specialists and neuropathologists is key. There is an increasing shift towards genetic testing as the initial diagnostic investigation of choice, as is already commonplace for McArdle disease (GSD type 5).

An electromyogram (EMG) and muscle biopsy (e.g. lack of myophosphorylase staining on muscle biopsy, suggesting McArdle disease) can yield important clues to help support a diagnosis of a specific metabolic myopathy or highlight clues to an alternative diagnosis mimicking a metabolic myopathy (e.g. myotonic discharges on EMG, which might suggest myotonic dystrophy).

An overview of the primary diseases to consider in adults

Glycogen storage disorders

During high intensity exercise, and particularly during activities which involve prolonged muscle contraction (e.g. weightlifting which causes muscle ischaemia), energy for myofibre contraction is supplied via anaerobic glycolysis (breakdown of glucose for the production of adenosine triphosphate [ATP]; see Figure 5.1). The glycogen storage disorders reflect defects in the metabolic pathways that store and mobilize glycogen (i.e. glycogenolysis, in order to produce glucose for glycolysis), or in some cases defects in the process of glycolysis itself, leading to inadequacy of carbohydrate metabolism to meet myofibre energy demand.

McArdle disease (GSD type 5)

Background

McArdle disease, first described by Dr Brian McArdle in 1951, is inherited in an autosomal recessive pattern and is the most common disorder of carbohydrate

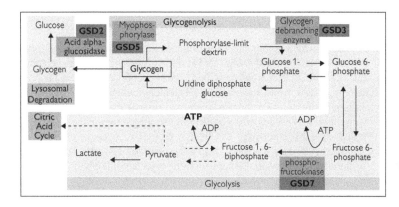

Figure 5.1 Summary of biochemical processes of glycogenolysis, glycolysis, and lysosomal degradation. Key glycogen storage disorders that can present in adulthood and associated enzymes are shown in shaded boxes. Dotted arrows represent omitted intermediate steps. GSD: glycogen storage disorder; ATP: adenosine triphosphate; ADP: adenosine diphosphate.

metabolism. McArdle disease occurs due to mutations in the *PYGM* gene, which encodes the skeletal muscle isoform of myophosphorylase. The cardiac and hepatic isoforms remain unaffected. Myophosphorylase is involved in converting glycogen to glucose 1-phosphate as part of glycogenolysis (Figure 5.1).

As a consequence of myophosphorylase deficiency, skeletal muscle fibres depend upon direct influx of glucose from the blood stream, or on other catabolic process (e.g. fatty acid or purine nucleotide metabolism) for energy production. Periods of relative muscle ischaemia (e.g. prolonged holding of heavy weights), predispose those with McArdle disease to developing myalgia and early fatigue of exercised muscles due to lack of immediately available systemic glucose to bypass the defective pathway. In the face of such exercise, a failure of lactate production is observed in tandem with an exaggerated hyperammonaemia, reflecting the defective glycolytic process and increasing reliance on alternative sources for ATP generation.

Clinical features

Symptoms of McArdle disease usually develop in childhood, although presentation may not be until early adulthood, and presentation in even late adulthood is well recognized. Males and females are equally affected. All patients will report exercise intolerance with many reporting post-exertional pigmenturia. The 'second wind' phenomenon, as described above, is reported in most patients. This recovery in function occurs due to increased cardiac output during exercise and an ensuing increased delivery of circulating glucose to muscle for use in glycolysis, without the need for glycogenolysis. Additionally, a more gradual increase in fatty acid metabolism occurs from breakdown of adipose and transportation of fatty acids to muscle for catabolism.

As muscle relaxation is also an energy dependent process, severe and prolonged painful muscle contractures can occur during and after exercise, leading to myonecrosis. Perhaps around one-third of patients, particularly those over 40 years of age, will develop fixed proximal upper limb and paraspinal muscle weakness.

McArdle disease shares clinical features with other glycogen storage disorders, especially Tarui disease (GSD type 7). It is difficult to distinguish between these disorders on clinical grounds alone, although there are sometimes features that can be used to help differentiate. For example, Tarui disease is associated with haemolytic anaemia due to involvement of phosphofructokinase isoforms in reticulocytes (reticulocyte count and/or serum bilirubin levels often raised).

Investigations

The CK level is usually raised, even after prolong periods of rest. However, a large variation in CK levels are seen and, occasionally, can be normal. Therefore, this investigation should not be used in isolation and further work-up should be performed in those with a suggestive clinical picture, even with a normal CK.

In the past, the forearm ischaemic lactate test (as originally described by McArdle) was used to confirm the diagnosis. A failure of exercise-associated lactate production in the face of normal or exaggerated ammonia production is the expected finding for McArdle disease. However, such exertion can induce painful muscle contractures or produce false negative (e.g. as a result of poor effort) or false positive (e.g. diagnosis may be an alternative enzyme defect producing same outcome) results. Thus, this test is now rarely performed, although supervised exercise testing to observe the 'second wind' phenomenon may be used and is useful for disease monitoring.

Muscle biopsy is also now less regularly performed, but will show increased Periodic Acid-Schiff (PAS) staining (reflecting increased levels of intramuscular glycogen, which cannot be catabolized) and an absence of myophosphorylase staining. Quantitative enzyme activity testing will show very low or undetectable residual activity.

Many now use genetic testing in the first instance in those with typical clinical features of McArdle disease. Practice varies between centres, but initially targeted mutation analysis may be performed looking for the most common mutations. In particular, the p.Arg50Ter (sometimes referred to as R50X) mutations of the *PYGM gene* can be found in up to 85% of Caucasian probands and p.Gly205Ser in up to a further 10%. If these are negative, then sequence analysis and deletion/duplication analysis may be required.

Therapy

Currently, treatment relies upon dietary modification (a mixture of 'background' complex carbohydrates with ingestion of 'simple' carbohydrates prior to exertion) and supervised aerobic exercise programmes. Patients should be advised to avoid anaerobic activity patterns, where isometric (static) or eccentric (lengthening) muscle contractions are frequent (e.g. weight training, squats). Involvement of a specialist metabolic multi-disciplinary team, including dieticians and physiotherapists is desirable.

Late-onset Pompe disease (GSD type 2)

Background

Pompe disease (also known as GSD type 2 and 'acid maltase deficiency') is also autosomal recessive and occurs due to *GAA* gene mutations coding for lysosomal acid alpha-glucosidase (acid maltase; see Figure 5.1). Defects in acid alpha-glucosidase function lead to toxic build-up of intra-lysosomal glycogen, thus initiating events that culminate in cell death. Early and late-onset forms of the disease exist, which approximately correlate with enzyme activity levels. In the most severe congenital cases of Pompe disease, there is practically no measurable enzyme activity, while in adult onset forms there is residual enzyme activity of at least 30%.

Clinical features

Proximal muscle weakness, particularly in the lower limbs, is the most common symptom of late-onset Pompe disease and may be accompanied by fatigue, myalgia, respiratory muscle, and facial muscle weakness. Patients can complain of exercise intolerance, but largely due to shortness of breath and fatigue.

Investigations

The serum CK may be raised up to 10× upper limit of normal, but can be within normal range. Muscle MRI can demonstrate the extent of affected musculature. Often a strikingly selective pattern of muscle atrophy and fatty replacement is seen, rather than the more general involvement seen in the IIM. The diagnosis of Pompe disease has become easier in recent years with advent of a dry blood spot (DBS) screening assay, which estimates residual enzyme activity.

Since the advent of enzyme replacement therapy for Pompe disease, a lower threshold for screening patients using DBS enzymology has been seen. In particular, there has been increased screening of patients with cryptogenic muscle disorders, which has led to an increased rate of diagnosis of late-onset Pompe disease.

Treatment

Enzyme replacement therapy is available for the treatment of Pompe disease and has been the subject of a number of clinical trials, particularly in childhood onset forms. However, the efficacy in adults with milder and more slowly progressive phenotypes is more variable, and remains the subject of ongoing assessment.

Fatty acid oxidation defects

Long chain fatty acids, the major fraction of fatty acids in circulation, represent a key energy source for muscle during periods of endurance exercise or in situations where efforts to spare glucose are being made, e.g. during fasting. However, unlike short and medium chain fatty acids (which are able to freely diffuse across membranes) long chain fatty acids require specific transporter proteins to traverse outer and inner mitochondrial membrane before they can be catabolized (Figure 5.2).

The FAODs can present similarly to McArdle disease, particularly in children. Key differences in clinical features include the *type* of exercise that will induce symptoms and *timing* of symptom onset (and CK elevations) in relation to exercise. In FAODs, symptoms generally come on after long periods of low intensity 'endurance' exercise. Myalgia can also persist for many days post-exercise. Additionally, periods of fasting (e.g. for religious reasons) and fever can predispose patients with FAODs to developing symptoms. CK elevations in response to an inciting event can be dramatic, often in to the many hundreds of thousands (IU/L), although inter-ictal CK is usually normal.

Carnitine palmitoyltransferase II deficiency

The most common FAOD encountered is carnitine palmitoyltransferase II (CPTII) deficiency, caused by mutations in the *CPT2* gene. CPTII deficiency is inherited in an autosomal recessive pattern, although with a male predominance. There are

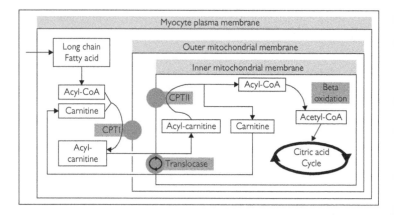

Figure 5.2 Summary of selected biochemical processes involved in fatty acid transport and oxidation. CPT: carnitine palmitoyltransferase; CoA: coenzyme A.

reports of disease manifesting heterozygotes, but thought to be rare. CPTII is a membrane protein located on the inner mitochondrial membrane, which plays a key role in the mitochondrial long chain fatty acid transportation system, which provides substrates for mitochondrial beta oxidation and the citric acid cycle (Figure 5.2).

There are childhood and adult onset forms of CPTII deficiency, which only partially correlate with severity of the genetic mutation. The childhood onset forms are multi-system disorders associated with liver failure and cardiomyopathy whereas the late-onset form is usually restricted to skeletal muscle.

Investigations will usually show an abnormal serum carnitine/acylcarnitine profile, with increased long-chain acylcarnitines. The CK can be markedly elevated (up to 400× the upper limit of normal) and can persist for some time after the inciting event. Confirmation of reduced CPTII enzyme activity can be demonstrated in muscle and other tissues, including cultured skin fibroblasts. However, such assays are difficult to perform and lack standardization between centres. Thus, diagnostic practice is now shifting towards earlier use of genetic testing. This may start with targeted analysis of more common genetic defects (e.g. p.Ser113Leu pathogenic variant found in 60% of those affected) before moving to more complex gene sequencing analysis.

Management of CPTII deficiency requires involvement of specialists in metabolic diseases, and an accompanying multidisciplinary team of dieticians and physiotherapists. In general, fasting periods should be minimized and a modified diet which contains reduced long chain fatty acids, and supplementation with medium chain fatty acids, which are free to diffuse across the mitochondrial membrane without involvement of defective pathways.

Table 5.1 Summary of a suggested clinical and therapeutic approach to patients presenting with symptoms suggestive of a metabolic myopathy

Detailed history	Exercise intolerance? Myalgia? Transient cramps? Second wind? Pigmenturia? Rhabdomyolysis? Family history (including consanguinity)? Patient with 'seronegative myositis' or 'treatment resistant myositis'?
Examination	Often normal, but look for fixed contractures and signs of mitochondrial disease (e.g. ptosis or ophthalmoplegia)

Further work-up

Where a metabolic myopathy is considered, early referral to specialist neuromuscular centre is advisable to facilitate further work-up

Initial investigations	May include: • Serum creatine kinase • Electromyography
Specialist investigations (may be performed in some cases according to the clinical presentation)	• Exercise testing, especially in those with suspected glycogen storage disorders • Serum carnitine/acylcarnitine profile for those with suspected fatty acid oxidation defects • Muscle biopsy, especially where there is concern about muscular dystrophy. With advancement in genetic testing, biopsy can be avoided in some cases • Enzyme activity testing (can be performed on dry blood spot, muscle biopsy, or from cultured skin fibroblasts)
Genetic analysis	• Presentation typical for McArdle disease (GSD type 5): in Caucasians, proceed to targeted mutation analysis (e.g. p.Arg50Ter) before more complex testing (gene sequencing, deletion/duplication analysis) • Presentation consistent with Pompe disease (GSD type 2): screen acid alpha glucosidase function by dry blood spot enzymology. If abnormal then proceed to genetic confirmation • Presentation consistent with fatty acid oxidation defect: targeted genetic analysis may be based on serum carnitine/acylcarnitine profile • Strategy varies between centres: early use of multigene panels is becoming more common. However, many patients will evade genetic confirmation of diagnosis even where the presentation is otherwise typical. Involvement of a genetic diagnostic service is important.

Management

Early involvement of a multidisciplinary team in a specialist neuromuscular centre is strongly recommended

Specific treatments	• Some diseases considered here (such as Pompe disease) have specific pharmacological treatments, which are now available • Dietary modification and supervised exercise programmes form part of the management of some metabolic myopathies. This should take place under direction of experienced dieticians and physiotherapists

Disorders of purine metabolism

Disorders of purine nucleotide metabolism may present with myalgia, fatigue, and exercise intolerance in adults. Infantile presentations with hypotonia are also described. The autosomal recessive myoadenylate deaminase deficiency (MADD) is the most common of these disorders. Most patients have a common mutation in the *AMPD1* gene and no adenosine monophosphate deaminase (APMPD) staining on muscle biopsy. Ribose supplements may help with muscle pain and fatigue, but will often induce diarrhoea.

Summary of approach to a patient with suspected metabolic myopathy

Metabolic myopathies and other genetic myopathies can clearly mimic IIM. Careful history taking can yield clues and certain 'red-flags' can be found on clinical examination that might highlight this possibility, or raise suspicion about other genetic myopathies. Where such 'red-flags' are encountered, use of immunosuppression should initially be withheld, unless IIM is strongly suspected. The diagnostic work-up and subsequent management of patients with metabolic myopathies is complex and early referral to a specialist neuromuscular centre is strongly recommended. A suggested clinical and therapeutic approach to such patients is summarized in Table 5.1.

SUGGESTED READING

Olpin SE, Murphy E, Kirk RJ, Taylor RW, Quinlivan R. (2015). The investigation and management of metabolic myopathies. *J Clin Pathol*; **68**(6): 410–17.

Quinlivan R, Buckley J, James M, et al. (2010). McArdle disease: a clinical review. *J Neurol Neurosurg Psychiatry*; **81**(11): 1182–8.

Scalco RS, Gardiner AR, Pitceathly RD, et al. (2015). Rhabdomyolysis: a genetic perspective. *Orphanet J Rare Dis*; **10**: 51.

Schoser B, Laforêt P, Kruijshaar ME, et al. (2015). 208th ENMC International Workshop: Formation of a European Network to develop a European data sharing model and treatment guidelines for Pompe disease Naarden, The Netherlands, 26–28 September 2014. *Neuromuscul Disord*; **25**(8): 674–8.

CHAPTER 6

Muscular dystrophies and other genetic myopathies

Stefen Brady and David Hilton-Jones

KEY POINTS

- Muscular dystrophies are a genetically heterogeneous group of muscle diseases characterized by progressive weakness and muscle wasting
- Some are multisystem disorders affecting the central nervous system, cardiovascular, endocrine, and gastrointestinal systems, in addition to skeletal muscle
- Careful clinical history and detailed physical examination remain the cornerstones of diagnosis, and guide molecular genetic testing
- Significant advances in molecular genetic testing means that a genetic diagnosis is now achievable for most patients with a muscular dystrophy
- Optimal management requires multi-speciality care

Introduction

Muscular dystrophies are a genetically and phenotypically heterogeneous group of progressive muscle diseases. The three commonest muscular dystrophies, in descending order, are myotonic dystrophy type I (DM1), the dystrophinopathies, including Duchenne muscular dystrophy (DMD) and Becker muscular dystrophy (BMD), and facioscapulohumeral muscular dystrophy (FSHD). Modern molecular genetic techniques have clarified the genetic mutations responsible for most muscular dystrophies. This has led to the discovery that mutations in different genes may cause an identical phenotype and that mutations within a single gene may result in different phenotypes. Therefore, despite advances in genetics, the importance of the clinical history and physical examination has increased rather than diminished. It is only through correctly identifying clinical features that clinicians can organize appropriate diagnostic investigations. Although muscular dystrophies are typically slowly progressive disorders where muscle atrophy and weakness are the defining characteristics, diagnostic confusion with IIM may still occur. For instance, a diagnosis of muscular dystrophy is considered only after failure of immunosuppressive treatment for a presumed case of IIM.

The myotonic dystrophies

Myotonic dystrophy type I (DM1, Steinert's disease, and dystrophia myotonica)

DM1 presents at any age from birth to late adulthood and affects the gastrointestinal, cardiac, endocrine, and central nervous systems. Its prevalence is around 3–15 per 100,000. DM1 is caused by an unstable and enlarged CTG repeat in the *DMPK* gene. The number of repeats correlates with disease severity and age of onset (Table 6.1). The enlarged CTG repeat expands further when transmitted to subsequent generations, potentially resulting in an earlier disease onset and more severe phenotype in affected children compared to the parents, a phenomenon known as 'genetic anticipation'. The DM1 phenotype depends on age of onset. With adult onset disease, the characteristic pattern of muscle involvement is facial, neck flexor, and distal limb weakness, with grip myotonia. In those with congenital onset disease, invariably transmitted by an affected mother rather than father, there is marked facial weakness, mild, but generalized limb weakness, and little or no myotonia in infancy. In those with congenital and childhood onset, learning difficulties and behavioural problems are usually prominent features.

Adult-onset patients have wasting of the temporalis and masseter muscles accompanied by facial weakness, ptosis, and weakness of neck flexion. Limb weakness is distal with finger flexion and ankle dorsiflexion particularly affected early on, but in later stages proximal muscles are also involved. Grip and percussion myotonia are present. Non-motor features include frontal balding and cataracts, which may be the only evidence of the condition in the transmitting parent with a smaller expansion of genetic repeats. Cardiac conduction defects, and arrhythmias and respiratory muscle weakness predisposing to chest infections, are the leading causes of death in DM1. The appropriate timing for insertion of a cardiac defibrillator or pacemaker is unknown. Excessive daytime sleepiness is

Table 6.1 Correlation between the size of the CTG repeat sequence in the *DMPK* gene and DM1 disease severity

Number of CTG repeats	Phenotype
<38	Normal
38–49	Premutation*
50–80	Mild DM1
100–1000	Classic (adult-onset) DM1
>1000	Congenital DM1

*Individuals harbouring 38–49 CTG repeats are asymptomatic, but the mutation may expand during transmission to subsequent generations.

common. Nocturnal hypoventilation and apnoea as a cause must be excluded, but in most patients excessive daytime sleepiness appears to be due to central mechanisms and as in narcolepsy, some patients respond to psychostimulant drugs such as modafinil. Gastrointestinal symptoms are reported by a third of patients, and abdominal pain, bloating, and episodic diarrhoea result in significant morbidity. Causes include bile acid malabsorption and small bowel bacterial overgrowth, which can be treated with cholestyramine or antibiotics. Endocrine problems in DM1 include gonadal insufficiency, insulin resistance (rarely diabetes), and hypothyroidism.

Creatine kinase (CK) is usually mildly raised, but can be normal. Electrophysiological assessment confirms the presence of myotonic discharges. Muscle biopsy is rarely performed, but shows dystrophic changes, type I muscle fibre atrophy, increased numbers of internal nuclei (more in type I fibres) and abnormal ring fibres. However, if clinically suspected the first investigation should be genetic testing, rendering other investigations as potentially unnecessary.

Management should include an annual clinical assessment to identify serious or disabling complications and an electrocardiogram, forced vital capacity measurement, and overnight oximetry if appropriate. Patients with cardiac symptoms should undergo cardiac assessment.

Myotonic dystrophy type 2 (proximal myotonic myopathy—PROMM)

Myotonic dystrophy type 2 (DM2) is characterized by proximal weakness, myotonia, and autosomal dominant inheritance without genetic anticipation. Onset is usually in middle age. Mild facial weakness is observed in two-thirds of patients. Myotonia is clinically less evident than in DM1, but may be detected on electromyography in some, but not all cases. Additional clinical features include cataracts (58%), myalgia (59%, leading some patients to be incorrectly diagnosed as having fibromyalgia), calf hypertrophy, tremor, hearing loss, endocrine disturbances including diabetes mellitus and infertility, and cardiac conduction abnormalities (13%). DM2 is milder than DM1 and hypersomnolence, dysphagia, and cognitive impairment are not seen. CK is mildly increased. Muscle biopsy may be normal or abnormal, with type II muscle fibre atrophy, increased numbers of internal nuclei (more in type II fibres) and abnormal ring fibres. The genetic mutation responsible is a CCTG repeat expansion in the *CNBP* (previously called *ZNF9*) gene.

Dystrophinopathies: Duchenne and Becker muscular dystrophy

The dystrophinopathies, which include DMD and the milder BMD are multisystem X-linked disorders due to mutations in the *DMD* gene, which encodes for the large dystrophin protein. DMD affects around 1:3500–1:6000 male births. The incidence of BMD is probably one-third that of DMD. Advances in management, particularly use of non-invasive ventilation, have led to a marked improvement in life-expectancy in DMD.

Boys with DMD present between 3 and 5 years of age with delayed motor milestones, toe walking, or difficulty running. Examination reveals calf hypertrophy, lordotic posture, and limb-girdle weakness. Non-progressive cognitive impairment affects one-third of patients and psychiatric problems are not uncommon. However, some individuals achieve high level academic success. Patients with DMD are wheelchair-dependent by around 12 years of age, whereas those with BMD remain ambulant at 16 years of age. Those who fall in-between these cut-offs are considered to have an intermediate form. Kyphoscoliosis is a common problem which adversely affects ventilatory function and respiratory insufficiency is one of the major causes of death in DMD. Eventually, nearly all patients with DMD develop cardiac disease. As respiratory management has improved and patients live longer the proportion dying from cardiac disease has increased.

Investigations show a markedly elevated CK. Muscle biopsy reveals dystrophic changes with muscle fibre necrosis and regeneration. Immunohistochemistry or immunoblotting for dystrophin are performed using antibodies to the protein C-terminal, N-terminal, and rod-domain. Approximately two thirds of genetic mutations causing DMD and BMD are large deletions. Up to one third of mutations arise *de novo*.

Patients with DMD have complex cardiorespiratory, endocrine, and orthopaedic care needs and require multi-speciality care. Corticosteroids (prednisolone and deflazacort) prolong ambulation, reduce the need for scoliosis surgery and help preserve cardiorespiratory function. The optimum duration of treatment and dosing regimen are uncertain. Molecular therapies are being developed and undergoing trials, including exon-skipping and the prevention of recognition of premature stop codons caused by nonsense mutations.

BMD has a milder phenotype and may not present until late adulthood. Other presentations of *DMD* mutations are isolated quadriceps weakness, myalgia and cramps, rhabdomyolysis, hyperCKaemia, and X-linked cardiomyopathy. Approximately 10% of female carriers are symptomatic; calf hypertrophy is common, severe proximal weakness is rare. Even in the absence of skeletal muscle involvement, some carriers may develop cardiomyopathy and should be offered regular cardiac screening.

Facioscapulohumeral muscular dystrophy

The prevalence of FSHD is approximately 5 per 100,000. It is an autosomal dominant disorder, but one-third of cases are due to *de novo* mutations. A total of 95% of cases are caused by a reduction in the D4Z4 repeat sequence on chromosome 4qA, referred to as FSHD1. The remainder are due to mutations in *SMCHD1* on chromosome 18, referred to as FSHD2.

The D4Z4 repeat sequence is found at three locations within the genome, however, FSHD1 is only associated with a truncated repeat sequence on chromosome 4qA. The deletion size loosely correlates with disease severity and age at onset: <10 kB (one to four repeats)—severe early onset disease, <35 kB (five to eight repeats)—classical FSHD, 35–38 kB (9–10 repeats)—is a grey area in which some individuals may be symptomatic.

FSHD is associated with a characteristic pattern of weakness, which is often asymmetric and progresses in a craniocaudal direction. Patients have weakness of eye closure and transverse smile, and may report difficulty whistling or using a straw. Scapular winging due to periscapular muscle weakness often brings an individual to medical attention. Scapular fixation surgery is considered on an individual basis. Deltoid muscle strength is preserved. Disproportionate atrophy of the clavicular head of pectoralis major and the upper arm muscles is visible. Biceps is the most frequently affected humeral muscle. Abdominal muscle weakness results in a protuberant abdomen, out of keeping with the rest of an individual's body habitus and marked lumbar lordosis. Beevor's sign, i.e. the abnormal upward movement of the umbilicus with neck flexion when supine, is a relatively specific and sensitive clinical sign for FSHD. Ankle dorsiflexion weakness can be the presenting feature, but facial or scapular weakness is usually present on examination. Individuals often complain of marked back or shoulder pain in the absence of significant weakness, the reasons for this are unknown.

Atypical presentations include absent or minimal facial weakness and camptocormia. Respiratory insufficiency affects <1% of patients. Extramuscular manifestations include sensorineural hearing loss and retinal vasculopathy (Coat's disease) in early-onset cases.

If FSHD is suspected clinically, then the first investigation should be genetic testing. Serum CK may be normal or moderately raised. Muscle biopsy can be normal or reveal rimmed vacuoles, inflammatory infiltrates, and increased major histocompatibility (MHC) class I staining. The latter is also typically observed in IIM.

Limb girdle muscular dystrophies

The ever increasing number of limb girdle muscular dystrophies (LGMD) means that a description of each individual disorder is beyond the scope of this chapter. For more detailed information the reader is directed to recent review articles and the Washington University Neuromuscular Disease Center website. LGMD are characterized by the presence of prominent shoulder girdle and pelvic girdle weakness. Eight autosomal dominant and 23 autosomal recessive LGMD have been described to date. The recessive LGMD are nine times more common than the dominant ones. Each LGMD disorder is denoted by the number 1 or 2 indicating dominant or recessive inheritance, respectively, and a capital letter signifies the order of discovery of the genetic mutation. For instance, LGMD1A represents the first autosomal dominant LGMD to be discovered, and which is caused by a mutation in *MYOT* encoding for the myofibrillar protein myotilin. Many LGMD are now more commonly referred to by the affected protein, e.g. myotilinopathy for LGMD1A and dysferlinopathy for LGMD2B.

Despite similarities between the LGMD, differences in age at onset, ethnic origin of patients, presence of cardiac or respiratory disease, examination findings, and investigation results inform the differential diagnosis and guide initial molecular genetic investigations. Distinctive features include selective muscle atrophy, such as gastrocnemius and biceps atrophy in dysferlinopathy (LGMD2B), muscle hypertrophy, including macroglossia observed in the sarcoglycanopathies (LGMD2C-F), and contractures that are prominent in laminopathy (LGMD1B).

The CK is often unhelpful, typically being mildly raised, although very high levels (>8000 IU/L) may be found in caveolinopathy (LGMD1C), calpainopathy (LGMD2A), dysferlinopathy (LGMD2B), sarcoglycanopathies (LGMD2C-F), anoctaminopathy (LGMD2L), and LGMD2I (Renard 2015). Findings on muscle biopsy with immunohistochemistry for sarcolemmal proteins and immunoblotting also provide important clues to the final diagnosis.

A recent study conducted across the North of England found that patients with LGMD accounted for 6.2% of a specialist neuromuscular clinic cohort. Over a quarter of the LGMD patients, the largest proportion, had calpainopathy (LGMD2A; Norwood et al. 2009). Similar findings have been reported in other studies across the world. It is important to note that despite detailed clinical assessments and thorough investigation, a precise genetic diagnosis is still not achieved in all LGMD patients.

Oculopharyngeal muscular dystrophy

Oculopharyngeal muscular dystrophy is a late onset autosomal dominant disease caused by a 12–17 GCN trinucleotide repeat sequence in *PABPN1*. Autosomal recessive cases are reported and can be more severe. Ptosis is usually the presenting symptom and occurs after 40 years of age. Additional features include ophthalmoparesis, dysphagia, and limb girdle weakness. Management includes ptosis surgery and either botulinum toxin injection, endoscopic dilatation, or cricopharyngeal myotomy for dysphagia. CK is mildly elevated. Rimmed vacuoles and 8.5-nm intranuclear tubulofilaments are observed on muscle biopsy. The characteristic clinical phenotype means that genetic testing is usually the first investigation performed.

Muscle dystrophies with marked joint contractures

Emery–Dreifuss muscular dystrophy

Emery–Dreifuss muscular dystrophy (EDMD) is characterized by early joint contractures, relatively mild weakness, and cardiac disease. Mutations in seven different genes are known to cause EDMD. Mutations in *EMD* and *LMNA* encoding inner nuclear membrane proteins emerin and lamin A/C are the commonest causes. Mutations in *EMD* cause X-linked (XL)-EDMD and mutations in *LMNA* result in autosomal dominant and rarely recessive EDMD.

Classic XL-EDMD is characterized by early joint contractures affecting elbows, Achilles tendons or spine, usually before 10 years of age. Humeroperoneal weakness is evident by the third decade. Cardiac disease is observed in most patients by 30 years of age, and includes arrhythmias, conduction abnormalities, and dilated cardiomyopathy. Infrequently, female carriers have clinically apparent disease. All female carriers should be assessed for cardiac disease. CK is moderately elevated and muscle biopsy reveals myopathic changes. In 95% of cases due to mutations in *EMD*, immunohistochemistry for emerin is absent, whereas emerin and lamin A/C staining are similar to normal controls in EDMD due to mutations in *LMNA*.

Autosomal dominant EDMD is clinically similar to XL-EDMD, but weakness may precede the onset of joint contractures, which are usually present before the 3rd decade. In addition to EDMD, mutations in *LMNA* cause dilated cardiomyopathy with conduction system disease, LGMD1B, Charcot-Marie-Tooth disease type 2, familial lipodystrophy, and progeria. These different conditions may coexist within the same family.

Collagen VI-related muscular dystrophies

The collagen VI-related disorders, autosomal recessive Ullrich congenital muscular dystrophy (UCMD) and the milder dominant Bethlem myopathy are characterized by weakness, joint contractures, and distal laxity, with cutaneous abnormalities. *De novo* mutations and autosomal dominant inheritance may also occur in UCMD.

The typical clinical picture of UCMD is neonatal onset generalized weakness, which is severe, proximal joint contractures, distal joint laxity, and skeletal abnormalities. Contractures may disappear early in disease and recur with increasing age. Weakness in Bethlem myopathy is proximal and joint contractures are distal, involving finger flexors, elbows, and ankles. Skin changes include keloid scarring and keratosis pilaris. Respiratory failure may occur in ambulant patients. Cardiac involvement has not been reported. Atypical presentations include weakness without contractures.

Investigations reveal a mildly elevated CK. In Bethlem myopathy, muscle magnetic resonance imaging (MRI) can show a peculiar pattern of central rectus femoris involvement. Imaging changes are more generalized in UCMD. Muscle biopsy is mildly myopathic. Immunohistochemistry for collagen VI is useful if demonstrably absent or markedly reduced, but it can be normal in Bethlem myopathy. Analysis of collagen VI production in fibroblasts from skin biopsy can be helpful.

Distal myopathies

The distal myopathies encompass a genetically heterogeneous group of disorders with preferential early involvement of distal limb muscles. Age at disease onset and pattern of weakness, CK, and muscle biopsy are useful for narrowing the differential diagnosis, see Table 6.2. Increasingly, MRI is being used to aid diagnosis. Myopathies such as DM1, FSHD, and EDMD may present with distal weakness. However, the presence of additional distinctive features on examination means these conditions rarely cause diagnostic difficulty.

The myofibrillar myopathies (MFM) and hereditary inclusion body myopathies (hIBM) may present as distal myopathies. MFM and hIBM share some pathological findings with sporadic inclusion body myositis (sIBM), namely rimmed vacuoles and eosinophilic inclusions. However, they are clinically quite different and the marked inflammatory infiltrates seen in sIBM are usually absent in these other conditions. The MFM are predominantly autosomal dominant, adult onset disorders grouped together on the basis of their pathological features of rimmed vacuoles and large congophilic inclusions, myofibrillar protein aggregates visible with immunohistochemistry, and myofibrillar disruption observed with electron microscopy. Currently, mutations in eight genes are known to cause MFM. Extramuscular manifestations include cardiomyopathy and cardiac conduction disturbances, respiratory insufficiency, cataracts, joint contractures, and neuropathy.

hIBM includes a diverse group of autosomal dominant/recessive disorders, though two conditions deserve specific mention. Autosomal recessive hIBM2 (also known as GNE myopathy, Nonaka myopathy, quadriceps sparing myopathy, and distal myopathy with rimmed vacuoles) is due to mutations in the *GNE* gene. Autosomal dominant inclusion body myopathy associated with Paget's disease of the bone and frontotemporal dementia (IBMPFD) is due to mutations in *VCP*. GNE myopathy is a distal myopathy with characteristic sparing of the quadriceps muscles and typically presents around the third decade. In IBMPFD the earliest and most frequent features are weakness (90%), and Paget's disease (50%) occurring in the 5th decade. Frontotemporal dementia occurs later and affects 30% of patients.

Differentiating the muscular dystrophies and the idiopathic inflammatory myopathies

In theory, differentiating muscular dystrophies and IIM should not pose a problem. The former are characterized by slowly progressive weakness and wasting over years, a distinctive pattern of weakness, a positive family history (sometimes), and a dystrophic muscle biopsy, whereas the latter are characterized by acute or subacute onset proximal weakness, muscle oedema on MRI and a florid inflammatory cell infiltrate on muscle biopsy. However, in practice, diagnosis can be difficult and sometimes a diagnosis of muscular dystrophy is only considered after a patient has failed to respond to several immunosuppressive treatments. Patients with a non-specific limb-girdle pattern of weakness of uncertain duration, or a muscle biopsy out-of-keeping with the clinical picture, often present the greatest diagnostic difficulty. Inflammation on muscle biopsy may be absent

Table 6.2 Clinical presentations, pathological features, and genotypes of the distal myopathies

Distal myopathy (aka)	Allelic disorders	Gene	Inheritance	Onset	Typical presentation	Additional clinical features	CK	Muscle biopsy	Distribution of affected muscles on MRI
Classic late-onset distal myopathies									
Welander myopathy		TIA1	AD	Late adulthood	Finger extension weakness	Uncommonly may present with ankle dorsiflexion weakness. Almost exclusively limited to Scandinavia.	–/+	Rimmed vacuoles may be seen	Anterior, posterior, and lateral lower leg
Udd myopathy (tibial muscular dystrophy)	HMERF LGMD2J CMD1G CMH9	TTN	AD	Late adulthood	Ankle dorsiflexion weakness	Early respiratory weakness. Almost exclusively limited to Finland.	–/+	Rimmed vacuoles	Anterior lower leg
Markesbury–Griggs (ZASPopathy)	MFM4 CMD1C CMH24	ZASP (LBD3)	AD	Late adulthood	Ankle dorsiflexion weakness	Cardiomyopathy	–/+	Rimmed vacuoles, eosinophilic inclusions, amyloid deposits, and IHC reveals myofibrillar aggregates	Posterior (medial gastrocnemius and soleus) lower leg

continued >

Table 6.2 Clinical presentations, pathological features, and genotypes of the distal myopathies (continued)

Distal myopathy (aka)	Allelic disorders	Gene	Inheritance	Onset	Typical presentation	Additional clinical features	CK	Muscle biopsy	Distribution of affected muscles on MRI
Classic early-onset distal myopathies									
Laing myopathy		MYH7	AD (de novo mutations in 1/3)	Childhood	Ankle dorsiflexion weakness	The combination of the hanging big toe sign, finger extension, and neck flexion weakness is said to be pathognomonic. Cardiomyopathy infrequently.	−/+	Hypotrophic type I muscle fibres	Anterior lower leg
Nonaka myopathy (hIBM2, DMRV, QSM, GNE myopathy)		GNE	AR	Early adulthood	Ankle dorsiflexion weakness	Quadriceps are rarely involved despite advanced weakness	+/ ++	Rimmed vacuoles	Anterior lower leg
Miyoshi myopathy	LGMD2B	DYS	AR	Early adulthood	Ankle plantarflexion weakness	Atrophy of biceps brachii	+++	Absent dysferlin IHC	Posterior lower leg

Others

I. Myofibrillar myopathies

	aka	Gene	Inheritance	Onset	Distal weakness	Other features	CK	Histology	MRI/leg pattern
Desminopathy (hIBM1)	LGMD1E MFM1	DES	AD (rare AR and sporadic cases)	Early–late adulthood	Distal lower leg weakness	Cardic involvement, respiratory insufficiency, cataracts, neuropathy, and joint contractures	–/+	Rimmed vacuoles, eosinophilic inclusions, amyloid deposits, and IHC reveals myofibrillar aggregates	Lateral lower leg more affected than anterior and posterior
Myotilinopathy	LGMD1A MFM3	MYOT	AD	Late adulthood	Distal lower leg weakness		–/+		Posterior lower leg
αB-crystallinopathy	MFM2	CRYAB	AD	Late adulthood	Distal lower leg weakness		–/+		Similar to desminopathy
Filaminopathy	MFM5	FLNC	AD	Late adulthood	Weakness of grip		–/+		Posterior or both posterior and anterior
2. IBMPFD		VCP	AD	Late adulthood	Onset may resemble Welander or Udd myopathies	Weakness may be limb girdle or scapuloperoneal. Extramuscular features include frontotemporal dementia and Paget's disease.	–/+	Rimmed vacuoles	Anterior
3. Anoctaminopathy (MMD3)	LGMD2L	ANO5	AR	Early adulthood	Ankle plantarflexion weakness	Often asymmetric calf involvement	+++		Posterior

aka, also known as; CK, creatine kinase; –/+, normal or mildly raised; +/++, mildly or moderately raised; +++, markedly raised; MRI, magnetic resonance imaging; AD, autosomal dominant; HMERF, hereditary myopathy with early respiratory failure; LGMD, limb girdle muscular dystrophy; CMD, congenital muscular dystrophy; CMH, familial hypertrophic cardiomyopathy; IHC, immunohistochemistry; AR, autosomal recessive; hIBM, hereditary inclusion body myopathy; DMRV, distal myopathy with rimmed vacuoles; QSM, quadriceps sparing myopathy; MFM, myofibrillar myopathy; IBMPFD, inclusion body myopathy associated with Paget's disease of the bone and frontotemporal dementia; MMD, Miyoshi muscular dystrophy.

in IIM and present in muscular dystrophies. The muscular dystrophies in which inflammatory infiltrates may be observed include: FSHD, dystrophinopathies, titinopathy, dysferlinopathy (LGMD2B), and GNE myopathy. Other investigations may also be misleading. MHC class I upregulation on muscle fibres is typically associated with IIM, but may also occur in many dystrophies. Irritative changes on electrophysiological assessment are usually considered as suggestive of an IIM, but can also be found in muscular dystrophies. Muscle oedema on MRI is typical for IIM, but may also be seen in muscular dystrophies. Fatty infiltration of muscles on MRI should raise suspicion that the diagnosis is likely to be that of a muscular dystrophy, however, this may also be found in longstanding IIM. Additional immunohistochemistry for sarcolemmal proteins, such as dysferlin, or immunoblotting may help.

In the majority of cases, a careful history and thorough examination leads to the correct diagnosis. Rarely do patients with muscular dystrophy report rapid disease progression. Myotonia, muscle atrophy and hypertrophy, distal weakness, asymmetry, joint contractures and laxity, and family history all suggest that the diagnosis is more likely to be a muscular dystrophy. The exception is sIBM, in which slowly progressive, asymmetric distal weakness is typical. If the diagnosis is still in doubt, clinicians are strongly advised to return to individual patients, and repeat the history and examination (Hilton-Jones 2014).

REFERENCES

Hilton-Jones D. (2014). Myositis mimics: how to recognize them. *Curr Opin Rheumatol*; **26**: 663–70.

Neuromuscular Disease Center. Website, Washington DC: Washington University. (accessed 29 August 2017).

Norwood FL, Harling C, Chinnery PF. (2009). Prevalence of genetic muscle disease in Northern England: in-depth analysis of a muscle clinic population. *Brain*; **132**: 3175–86.

Renard D. (2015). Serum CK as a guide to the diagnosis of muscle disease. *Pract Neurol*; **15**: 121.

CHAPTER 7

Evaluation of hyperCKaemia

Andrew L. Mammen and Jessica R. Nance

KEY POINTS

- Causes of elevated creatine kinase (CK) levels include myositis, infection, certain medication exposure, illicit substance exposure, endocrine/electrolyte abnormalities, and inherited muscle diseases
- In the evaluation of HyperCKaemia, physicians should prioritize the identification of reversible causes
- If no clearly reversible cause of hyperCKaemia is identified, additional investigations such as electromyography, muscle biopsy, and genetic testing may assist in identification of a responsible etiology
- In some cases, extensive evaluation of hyperCKaemia fails to reveal an etiology

---

Introduction

Creatine kinase (CK) is an intracellular enzyme, so normally only low levels are released into the bloodstream with transient sarcolemmal disruptions that occur with routine daily activities. Following an acute muscle injury, serum CK levels rise within 2–12 hours, peaking 3–5 days post-injury, then declining over the subsequent 6–10 days. When muscle injury is ongoing, elevated CK levels will be sustained. While normal serum CK levels are often considered to be <200 U/L, CK values are often higher in men compared with women and, more significantly, in black compared with white individuals (George 2016); indeed, up to 2.5% of healthy black men may have a CK ≥1000 IU/L.

Many acquired and inherited conditions may cause disruption of skeletal muscle cell membranes, with resulting leakage of CK from affected muscle cells, and subsequent elevation of serum CK levels. For example, myotoxic medications may cause muscle cell necrosis by mechanisms often poorly understood. Alternatively, inherited deficiencies of metabolic enzymes can result in exercise-induced adenosine triphosphate (ATP) depletion, with subsequent myofibre necrosis. In other cases, muscle membrane repair processes are unable to keep up with activity-induced muscle fibre damage, as occurs in some inherited muscular dystrophies. This limits efficient repair of damaged muscle membranes, so causing a chronic leakage of CK from damaged muscle cells.

Elevations in serum CK can present acutely, sub-acutely, or chronically. When symptoms of muscle pain, weakness, and CK levels >1000 IU/L present over the course of a few days (or shorter time period), the diagnosis of rhabdomyolysis can be made. In these circumstances, patients often describe dark urine due to increased urinary myoglobin concentrations. An inciting physical activity stimulus may be elicited from the history or exam, helping to guide diagnostic evaluation and allowing for prevention of future episodes. Alternatively, the patient may present with a subacute or chronic onset of muscle symptoms.

Causes of creatine kinase elevation

Acquired hyperCKaemia

Myositis

The idiopathic inflammatory myopathies are an important cause of acquired muscle injury presenting with elevated serum CK. The degree of CK elevation in dermatomyositis and polymyositis is highly variable, ranging from being within the normal range to >100,000 IU/L in occasional cases. The peak CK level in patients with any immune-mediated necrotizing myopathy is almost always >1000 IU/L. However, CK levels may be substantially lower during early phases of disease. All forms of myositis can present with a fulminant picture, with features of rhabdomyolysis including acute weakness, muscle pain, and CK elevations >1,000 IU/L. The presence of rash, interstitial lung disease, or myositis-specific autoantibodies may help identify an autoimmune process as the cause of rhabdomyolysis. CK levels in inclusion body myositis are commonly less than 1,000 IU/L.

Infections

Viral infections, most often with influenza A or B, are a common cause of elevated CK, especially in children. Muscle pain, weakness, and elevated CK levels typically present towards the end of illness as the extramuscular viral symptoms are resolving. Other viral infections associated with rhabdomyolysis include Coxsackie virus, Epstein-Barr virus, cytomegalovirus, echovirus, herpes simplex virus, adenovirus, HIV and dengue.

Medications

Prescription medications may occasionally cause acute or sub-acute increases in serum CK levels. A list of medications associated with rhabdomyolysis is detailed in Box 7.1. Statins, especially in combination with certain CYP450-inhibitors, have been associated with muscle pain and weakness, and more rarely, with elevated CK levels. Acute rhabdomyolysis is rare, estimated to occur in less than 1 per 10,000 person-years. The risk of statin-associated myopathy is increased in older patients and those with a history of systemic illness, major surgery, hypothyroidism, and/or hepatic disease (Mammen and Amato 2010).

Box 7.1 Selected medications associated with rhabdomyolysis

- Aminocaproic acid
- Antidepressants causing serotonin syndrome
- Antihistamines
- Antipsychotics causing neuroleptic malignant syndrome
- Anti-retrovirals
  - Tenofovir/abicavir
  - Raltegravir
- Colchicine
- Colchicine + clarithromycin
- Colchicine + ciclosporin/tacrolimus
- Daptomycin
- Valproate semisodium
- Interferon alfa
- Lithium
- Ofloxacin/levofloxacin
- Statins (increased risk with hypothyroidism, certain genetic polymorphisms, liver disease, and diabetes)
  - Statins + fibrates
  - Statin + CYP450 inhibitors
  - Statin + CYP3A4 inhibitors
    - Diltiazem/amiodarone/verapamil
    - Macrolide antibiotics (erythromycin/clarithromycin)
    - Protease inhibitors
    - Sitagliptin
    - Colchicine
  - Statin + daptomycin
  - Statin + fluconazole
  - Statin + tacrolimus/cyclosporine

Adapted from Nance JR, Mammen AL (2015). Diagnostic evaluation of rhabdomyolysis. *Muscle Nerve*; 51: 793–810, with permission from John Wiley and Sons.

Antipsychotic medications are also associated with increased risk of muscle injury, often in the setting of neuroleptic malignant syndrome (Packard et al. 2014).

Drugs and illicit substances

Patients who abuse alcohol and illicit substances are at increased risk for muscle injury. In one study of 77 hospitalized patients with CK levels greater than 500 U/L, 80% had a history of acute or chronic alcohol and/or illicit drug use (Gabow et al. 1982). Muscle injury often presents acutely in such patients, thought to be related to direct muscle toxicity from the substances or their additives. In addition, increased sympathomimetic stimulation, as can be seen with ecstasy or lysergic acid diethylamide, may lead to muscle damage.

Toxins

Rarely, acute elevations of CK can be seen following exposure to poison or venoms. Snake, wasp, and spider venoms have all been associated with rhabdomyolysis. The mechanism of venom-induced muscle damage is thought to be related to direct muscle toxicity and/or muscle ischaemia in the setting of an induced coagulopathy. Ingestion of certain mushrooms is also associated with rhabdomyolysis. Rhabdomyolysis has also been reported following ingestion of European quails that feed on Hemlock seeds, or with ingestion of an unidentified toxin found in buffalo fish.

Electrolyte endocrine abnormalities

Muscle injury with elevated CK can also occur in patients with electrolyte disturbances, such as hyperkalaemia, hypophosphataemia, hypernatraemia, and hyponatraemia. These abnormalities may occur in the context of substance abuse, diabetes, or other endocrine disorders. Thyroid dysfunction, adrenal insufficiency, diabetes insipidus, and pituitary dysfunction have all been implicated as potential causes of acutely elevated CK levels. Hypokalaemia seen with inherited or acquired renal tubular dysfunction may also present with acutely elevated CK levels.

Sickle cell disease

Elevated CK levels and rhabdomyolysis have been described in patients with sickle cell disease. This is thought to be related to muscle ischaemia associated with intravascular coagulation, which can occur in the setting of illness, stress, dehydration, or metabolic acidosis (Devereux and Knowles 1985).

Benign exertional rhabdomyolysis

In certain apparently healthy patients with recurrent acute CK elevations associated with muscle pain and weakness, no cause of rhabdomyolysis can be identified. These episodes are often triggered by intense exercise, and may be influenced by race, gender, and level of physical fitness (Meltzer 1971; Alpers and Jones 2010). More recently, several single nucleotide polymorphisms have been identified, which are associated with development of benign exertional rhabdomyolysis (Deuster et al. 2013).

Genetic causes of hyperCKaemia

Metabolic myopathies

CK elevations in metabolic myopathies are most frequently observed after exercise, but may also be triggered by illness, fasting, or stress (see Chapter 5).

Practical approach to patient with hyperCKaemia

Evaluating patients with hyperCKaemia can be challenging and there is no 'one-size-fits-all' method for arriving at a definitive diagnosis. First, we suggest to determine whether an affected patient has likely had an acute rise in CK levels (i.e. rhabdomyolysis), or instead had a more chronic elevation in enzyme levels. Secondly, the authors suggest determining whether an affected patient is symptomatic with regard to muscle weakness or not. Based on these clinical features, they suggest differing approaches for evaluating patients with rhabdomyolysis (Figure 7.1), symptomatic chronic hyperCKaemia (Figure 7.2), and asymptomatic chronic hyperCKaemia (Figure 7.3).

Acute onset of elevated creatine kinase and muscle symptoms

When patients present with acute onset of weakness, muscle pain, muscle swelling, and/or dark urine that is accompanied by elevated CK levels, we suggest following the algorithm for evaluation of rhabdomyolysis (Figure 7.1). The history and examination should first be directed at identifying acquired and reversible causes, such as trauma, infection, medication exposure, autoimmune muscle disease, and alcohol/drug/toxin exposure. Initial screening of thyroid function and serum electrolytes can help to identify endocrine/electrolyte abnormalities.

Next, a history of preceding exercise or abnormally strenuous activity should be elicited. Symptom onset early after low-level exercise is characteristic of mitochondrial disorders. Muscle symptoms that occur only after intense activity suggest a disorder of glycogen metabolism. Confirming the onset of symptoms as being after submaximal activity, fasting, or illness is more likely in those with disorders of fatty acid oxidation. When a patient presents with a classic pattern suggestive of a metabolic myopathy, such as a history of the second wind phenomenon in myophosphorylase deficiency, then we recommend proceeding directly with genetic testing. In less obvious cases, a muscle biopsy may be helpful. However, we recommend avoiding muscle biopsy very soon after the acute presentation of rhabdomyolysis, as features of myonecrosis may obscure histologically characteristic evidence of a metabolic myopathy. We thus suggest waiting for 2 months before performing a diagnostic muscle biopsy. An exception to this general rule would be when an autoimmune myopathy is suspected. For example, in a patient without a definitive rash, perifascicular atrophy would be diagnostic of dermatomyositis, and lead to immediate treatment with immunosuppressive therapy.

If muscle biopsy does not suggest a metabolic myopathy, but does show other myopathic features (e.g. round atrophic fibres, fibrosis), then the possibility of inherited muscular dystrophy or congenital myopathy should be considered (see Chapter 6). Only if there are no histological abnormalities or definitive gene mutations should the diagnosis of 'benign rhabdomyolysis' be considered.

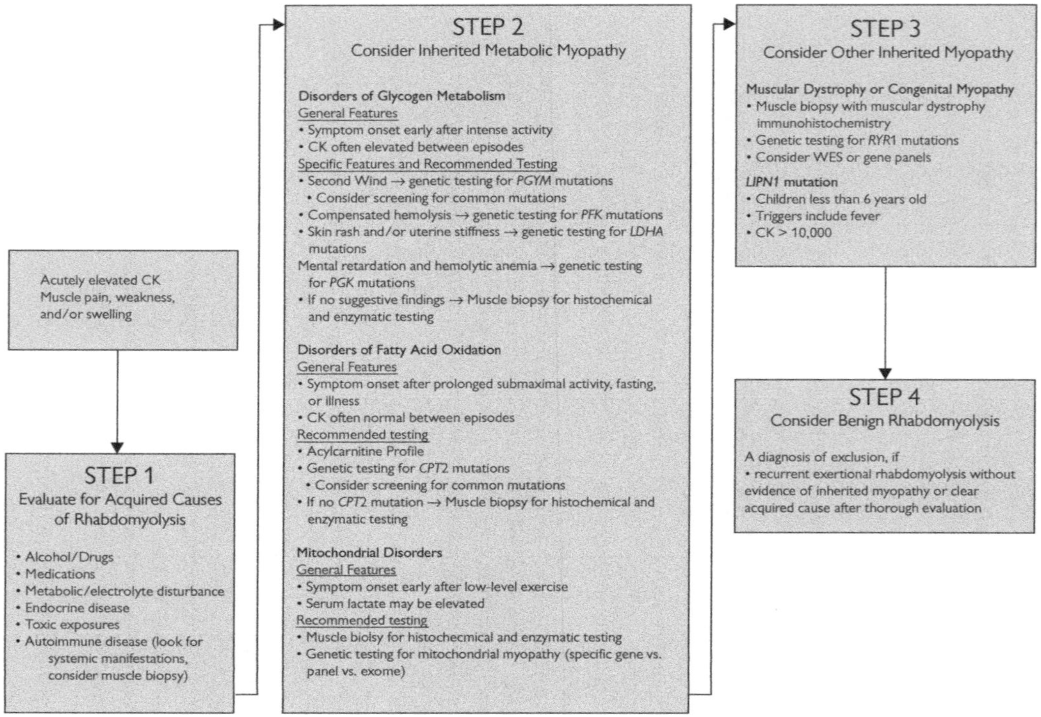
Acutely elevated CK
Muscle pain, weakness, and/or swelling
STEP 1
Evaluate for Acquired Causes of Rhabdomyolysis
• Alcohol/Drugs
• Medications
• Metabolic/electrolyte disturbance
• Endocrine disease
• Toxic exposures
• Autoimmune disease (look for systemic manifestations, consider muscle biopsy)
STEP 2
Consider Inherited Metabolic Myopathy
Disorders of Glycogen Metabolism
General Features
• Symptom onset early after intense activity
• CK often elevated between episodes
Specific Features and Recommended Testing
• Second Wind → genetic testing for PGYM mutations
• Consider screening for common mutations
• Compensated hemolysis → genetic testing for PFK mutations
• Skin rash and/or uterine stiffness → genetic testing for LDHA mutations
Mental retardation and hemolytic anemia → genetic testing for PGK mutations
• If no suggestive findings → Muscle biopsy for histochemical and enzymatic testing
Disorders of Fatty Acid Oxidation
General Features
• Symptom onset after prolonged submaximal activity, fasting, or illness
• CK often normal between episodes
Recommended testing
• Acylcarnitine Profile
• Genetic testing for CPT2 mutations
• Consider screening for common mutations
• If no CPT2 mutation → Muscle biopsy for histochemical and enzymatic testing
Mitochondrial Disorders
General Features
• Symptom onset early after low-level exercise
• Serum lactate may be elevated
Recommended testing
• Muscle biolsy for histochecmical and enzymatic testing
• Genetic testing for mitochondrial myopathy (specific gene vs. panel vs. exome)
STEP 3
Consider Other Inherited Myopathy
Muscular Dystrophy or Congenital Myopathy
• Muscle biopsy with muscular dystrophy immunohistochemistry
• Genetic testing for RYR1 mutations
• Consider WES or gene panels
LIPN1 mutation
• Children less than 6 years old
• Triggers include fever
• CK > 10,000
STEP 4
Consider Benign Rhabdomyolysis
A diagnosis of exclusion, if
• recurrent exertional rhabdomyolysis without evidence of inherited myopathy or clear acquired cause after thorough evaluation

Figure 7.1 Suggested evaluation of rhabdomyolysis.

Reproduced from Nance JR and Mammen AL (2015). Diagnostic evaluation of rhabdomyolysis. *Muscle Nerve*; 51: 793–810, with permission

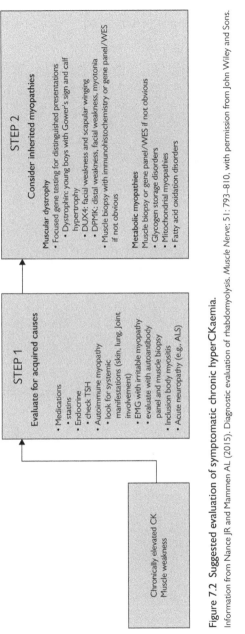

Figure 7.2 Suggested evaluation of symptomatic chronic hyperCKaemia.

Information from Nance JR and Mammen AL (2015). Diagnostic evaluation of rhabdomyolysis. *Muscle Nerve*; 51: 793–810, with permission from John Wiley and Sons.

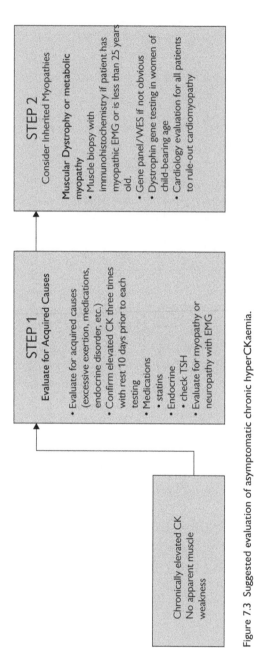

Figure 7.3 Suggested evaluation of asymptomatic chronic hyperCKaemia.

Adapted from Nance JR and Mammen AL (2015). Diagnostic evaluation of rhabdomyolysis. *Muscle Nerve*; 51: 793–810, with permission from John Wiley and Sons.

Chronically elevated CK
No apparent muscle
weakness

STEP 1

Evaluate for Acquired Causes

- Evaluate for acquired causes (excessive exertion, medications, endocrine disorder, etc.)
- Confirm elevated CK three times with rest 10 days prior to each testing
  - Medications
    - statins
  - Endocrine
    - check TSH
- Evaluate for myopathy or neuropathy with EMG

STEP 2

Consider Inherited Myopathies

Muscular Dystrophy or metabolic myopathy
- Muscle biopsy with immunohistochemistry if patient has myopathic EMG or is less than 25 years old.
- Gene panel/WES if not obvious
- Dystrophin gene testing in women of child-bearing age
- Cardiology evaluation for all patients to rule-out cardiomyopathy

Chronic elevation of serum creatine kinase with muscle symptoms

As in patients with rhabdomyolysis, those with more chronic CK elevations associated with muscle pain and/or weakness should first be evaluated for an acquired and potentially reversible cause of muscle damage (Figure 7.2). In addition to toxic medications and endocrine abnormalities, autoimmune myopathy should be considered. Associated clinical features such as rash, interstitial lung disease, and arthritis should prompt consideration of an autoimmune diagnosis. When the latter is suspected, a myositis antibody panel searching for myositis-specific/associated autoantibodies can aid in the diagnosis, and may help guide specific treatments. Additionally, muscle biopsy should be considered in these patients; as this may show characteristic findings of primary inflammation, myonecrosis, and/or perifascicular atrophy.

Inclusion body myositis (IBM) is another inflammatory myopathy that can present with chronic elevation of CK and progressive weakness (see Chapter 11). Electromyography may be helpful in distinguishing IBM from neurogenic causes of distal muscle weakness, some of which can cause marked CK elevations. For example, some patients with amyotrophic lateral sclerosis can present with CK levels >1000 IU/L, especially early during the course of especially aggressive disease.

When medications, endocrine dysfunction, autoimmune myopathy, IBM, and neurogenic causes have been excluded, one should consider a diagnosis of a muscular dystrophy or, rarely, a metabolic myopathy. There are many different types of rare inherited muscle diseases, so arriving at the correct diagnosis can be challenging. However, in many cases, the pattern of weakness or other clinical features may suggest a specific diagnosis (see Chapter 6).

In patients with clinical features typical of a specific disease, targeted genetic testing for the suspected gene defect should be performed where available. Otherwise, patients with suspected dystrophies or metabolic myopathies should be referred to specialist rheumatology or neurology clinics with extensive neuromuscular experience in diagnosing such patients. In addition, since patients with genetic disease affecting skeletal muscles may also have cardiac involvement, a screening electrocardiogram and echocardiogram are recommended in those with confirmed or suspected dystrophy.

Asymptomatic chronic hyperCKaemia

There is a population of patients with chronically elevated CK levels, but in whom no muscle signs or symptoms are present. As with all patients presenting with hyperCKaemia, their evaluation should similarly begin with a consideration of acquired causes. Once these have been ruled-out, the CK should be checked on two or three additional occasions after rest over 10 days prior to CK testing. If the CK remains elevated, the possibility of a mild or early inherited myopathy should be considered. In such cases, muscle biopsy may be revealing, e.g. in a population of 114 patients with elevated CK, and no or minimal muscle symptoms, 70 had normal muscle biopsies, but 44 had pathological changes present (Prelle et al. 2002). Among those with abnormal muscle biopsies, numerous diagnoses were eventually confirmed, including dystrophinopathy, limb-girdle muscular dystrophies, desminopathy, central core myopathy, tubular aggregate myopathy, and partial carnitine palmitoyl transferase type II deficiency. Nonetheless, in a significant proportion of patients with asymptomatic hyperCKaemia, no diagnosis will be found. In such patients, a diagnosis of benign hyperCKaemia will be made.

Women with CK levels greater than three times the upper limit of normal should be offered DNA testing to evaluate their carrier status for a dystrophin mutation. Those women of child-bearing age who harbour such a mutation should be counselled about the possibility of delivering a boy with Duchene or Becker's muscular dystrophy. Because cardiomyopathy may be associated with many of the genetic muscle diseases outlined previously, we recommend that patients with asymptomatic, chronic hyperCKaemia should also undergo screening electrocardiograhy and echocardiography.

Rarely, patients with chronically elevated CK levels and no apparent myopathy symptoms are found to have elevated macro-CK on CK electrophoresis. Elevation of type I macro-CK may be an indication of an underlying autoimmune process, while elevation of type II macro-CK may be associated with malignancy (Lee et al. 1994).

Summary

There are many potential causes of hyperCKaemia. In all patients with acute and chronic CK elevations, the immediate focus should be on identifying reversible causes. These include medication exposures, electrolyte/endocrine abnormalities, and autoimmune myopathy. Once these causes have been excluded, consideration should be given to inherited causes of muscle damage. We have provided guidelines for investigating for these causes and tailored this to streamline the process depending on whether the CK elevations are acute or chronic, and whether or not patients have muscle symptoms such as weakness. We expect these guidelines to aid in the diagnosis of patients with hyperCKaemia. However, it should be noted that a definitive diagnosis may not be reached even after a careful and comprehensive evaluation. If an obvious cause for CK elevation is not easily apparent, an early referral to a tertiary centre regularly dealing with muscle problems is recommended.

SUGGESTED READING

Alpers JP, Jones LK, Jr. (2010). Natural history of exertional rhabdomyolysis: a population-based analysis. *Muscle Nerve*; **42**(4): 487–91.

Deuster PA, Contreras-Sesvold CL, O'Connor FG, et al. (2013). Genetic polymorphisms associated with exertional rhabdomyolysis. *Eur J Appl Physiol*; **113**(8): 1997–2004.

Devereux S, Knowles SM. (1985). Rhabdomyolysis and acute renal failure in sickle cell anaemia. *Br Med J (Clin Res Ed)*; **290** (6483), 1707.

Gabow PA, Kaehny WD, Kelleher SP. (1982). The spectrum of rhabdomyolysis. *Medicine (Baltimore)*; **61**(3): 141–52.

George MD, Neilia-Kay M, Baker JF. (2016). Creatine kinase in the U.S. population: Impact of demographics, comorbidities, and body composition on the normal range. *Medicine;* **95**:33(e4344)

Lee KN, Csako G, Bernhardt P, Elin RJ. (1994). Relevance of macro creatine kinase type 1 and type 2 isoenzymes to laboratory and clinical data. *Clin Chem*; **40**(7 Pt 1): 1278–83.

Mammen AL, Amato AA. (2010). Statin myopathy: a review of recent progress. *Curr Opin Rheumatol*; **22**(6): 644–50.

Packard K, Price P, Hanson A. (2014). Antipsychotic use and risk of rhabdomyolysis. *J Pharm Pract*; **27**(5): 501–12.

Prelle A, Tancredi L, Sciacco M, et al. (2002). Retrospective study of a large population of patients with asymptomatic or minimally symptomatic raised serum creatine kinase levels. *J Neurol*; **249**(3): 305–11.

Important disease subtypes and associations

CHAPTER 8

Association with malignancy

Albert Selva-O'Callaghan and Ernesto Trallero-Araguás

KEY POINTS

- The temporal criterion (cancer and myositis diagnosed within 3 years) is the most important criterion for considering cancer-associated myositis
- The risk of cancer-associated myositis is higher in patients with dermatomyositis than in those with other types of myositis
- Positron emission tomography (PET)/computed tomography (CT) examination and anti-TIFIγ analysis should be considered as part of standard cancer screening for adult patients with dermatomyositis
- The outcome of patients with paraneoplastic dermatomyositis is more dependent on the cancer than on the myositis
- Cancer and myositis do not always run in parallel, and several scenarios are possible.

Introduction

Incidence of malignancy in different myositis subgroups

A population-based study involving a large cohort of patients with polymyositis (PM) and dermatomyositis (DM) recorded in a nationwide registry in Sweden and a study in patients with biopsy-proven disease in Australia, confirmed the association between cancer and inflammatory myopathies. The studies showed that the risk of cancer is higher in patients with DM than in those with PM, and that the association with sporadic inclusion body myositis is probably casual. The data indicated that the relative risk of cancer in DM patients is 3.4-fold higher than in the general population in women and 2.4-fold higher in men, and that the risk is somewhat lower in PM patients (1.7-fold greater in women and 1.8 in men). These results have been replicated in analyses of biopsy-proven myositis patients in other continents. Although it has long been suspected that patients with immune-mediated necrotizing myopathy are prone to cancer, large epidemiologic studies to support this association are lacking.

Several types of neoplastic diseases have been reported in association with myositis, with adenocarcinoma of the ovaries, breast, and gastrointestinal tract (gastric, colorectal, and pancreatic) being the most frequent. It is remarkable that almost any type of cancer can be involved, a clue to understanding the pathogenesis of the association. One paradigmatic example is the case of naso-pharyngeal carcinoma, relatively common in the Asian community, and the most highly represented myositis-associated cancer in a nationwide epidemiologic study conducted in China.

Although immunosuppressive therapy is usually administered to treat myositis and has been occasionally implicated in the development of cancer, available data do not support a clear drug-related association.

Risk factors for associated malignancy and screening approach

Given the fact that nearly one third of patients with myositis and particularly those with DM have a paraneoplastic condition, it seems logical to exclude occult neoplasm in patients who show no evidence of cancer at the time of the myositis diagnosis. Surprisingly, there remains no consensus regarding the intensity or peri-odicity of screening. Several risk factors for the development of malignant disease have been reported: older age, male gender, dysphagia, severe cutaneous mani-festations (necrosis or vasculitis), rapid-onset myositis, and elevated acute-phase reactant parameters (C-reactive protein and erythrocyte sedimentation rate) are all factors associated with higher malignancy risk. By contrast, interstitial lung dis-ease, Raynaud's phenomenon, and anti-synthetase antibodies (mainly anti-Jo1), are associated with lower risk of malignancy. Although these data are of value, they have lost some value (at least in relation to DM, the idiopathic inflammatory myopathy (IIM) most commonly associated with cancer) since identification of an autoantibody against transcriptional intermediary factor 1-gamma (anti-TIF1γ antibody), formerly named *anti-p155 antibody* or *anti-p155/140 antibody*. Since Targoff's initial description of this new autoantibody in myositis, observations of an association between anti-TIF1γ and malignancy in DM patients have prompted a meta-analysis of published studies: DM patients testing positive for anti-TIF1γ antibody have a very much higher risk of having cancer-associated myositis than those who are anti-TIF1γ negative.

A reasonable approach for occult malignancy screening in patients with myo-sitis includes a comprehensive clinical history (including the family history of colon cancer) thorough clinical examination, complete blood count, and exten-sive biochemistry analyses. Physicians should have a high degree of suspicion for the presence of cancer. For example, the presence of iron deficiency anaemia should lead to study of the gastrointestinal tract with gastroscopy and colon-oscopy. Analysis of tumour markers (CA 19-9 and CarcinoEmbtyonic Antigen [CEA]) should be routinely requested, and prostate-specific antigen (PSA) in men and ovarian markers (CA125) in women should also be requested. A com-prehensive radiologic approach is recommended, including mammography and gynaecological ultrasound study in women, and chest and abdominal computed tomography (CT) scanning in all patients. Urinary cytology is also required.

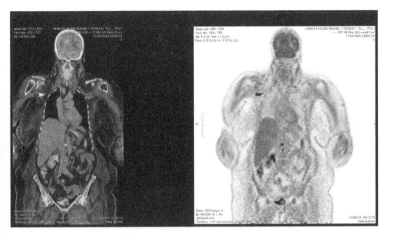

Figure 8.1 PET/CT images in a 67-year-old woman with refractory DM disclosed high uptake of lymphadenopathy at the upper and lower the diaphragm (SUVmax 23), suggestive of high-grade lymphoma, later confirmed by pathology. See Colour Plate Section.

One report has described the usefulness of whole-body [18F] fluorodeoxy-glucose positron emission tomography/computed tomography (FDG-PET/CT) for diagnosing occult malignant disease in patients with myositis. Although the diagnostic performance is similar to that of comprehensive conventional cancer screening, PET/CT has the advantage that only a single test is needed, making it a more convenient approach for the patient (Figure 8.1).

The recently described anti-TIFIγ antibodies, with a high negative predictive value for the detection of occult malignancy in patients with DM, will almost certainly have a major role in general screening of DM patients. Anti-TIFIγ can now be easily detected by relatively simple techniques, such as ELISA and immunoblotting, at a sensitivity and specificity similar to that achieved by immunoprecipitation, a much more complex and less widely available technique. Other autoantibodies, such as anti-NXP2, may also be associated with malignancy in myositis patients, although current evidence for such an association is limited. A proposed algorithm for cancer screening and follow-up in patients with myositis is described in Figure 8.2.

Links and relationships between cancer and myositis (pathophysiology)

Several studies have looked into the mechanisms of the relationship between cancer and myositis. Molecular mimicry, a cross-reaction between certain cancer

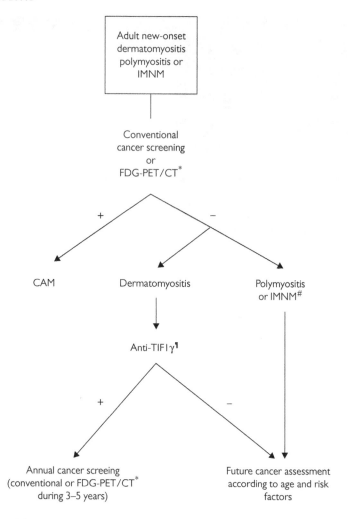

Figure 8.2 Algorithm for cancer screening in patients with idiopathic inflammatory myopathy.

IMNM, immuno-mediated necrotizing myopathy; FDG-PET/CT, [18F] fluorodeoxyglucose PET/computed tomography; CAM, cancer-associated myositis

* If available

¶ Association of anti-NXP2 with cancer needs further investigation.

In IMNM patients, one study has suggested a possible association between the presence of anti-HNGCoA autoantibodies and cancer. This theory needs further investigation.

antigens and myositis-specific antigens, has been demonstrated. As an example, Mi-2 (a specific myositis antigen) is overexpressed in certain lung and breast cancers, prompting a new theory to explain cancer-associated myositis. According to this concept, the immune system attacks the neoplasm and, unintentionally, also the muscle tissue. Some researchers have argued that a subset of patients with myositis (especially those with DM) should be viewed as 'cancer survivors' who never develop cancer because of effective surveillance of their immune system, but which is also responsible for the clinical presentation of DM.

Recent advances in our knowledge of the relationship between cancer and myositis, including identification of anti-TIFIγ antibody, are contributing to clarify this perplexing association. The precise role of anti-TIFIγ in the relationship between cancer and DM is not fully understood, but some lines of evidence support its participation as a link between the two disorders. TIFIγ overexpression was recently demonstrated in muscle regenerating cells, indicating a possible role similar to that mentioned for other myositis-specific antigens, e.g. Mi-2. Several hypotheses, such as the existence of a self-mutated TIFIγ wild-type protein, overexpression of TIFIγ protein in some types of cancer, and the presence of TIFIγ gene mutations in neoplastic cells have been suggested to explain the development of an immune reaction against this protein, expressed as anti-TIFIγ antibodies. At least one TIFIγ mutation (TRIM33: NM_015906:exon20: c. A3215G: p. Y1072C) has been found in a single DM patient with anti-TIFIγ antibodies and diagnosed with oat cell lung carcinoma (unpublished personal observation).

The link between TIFIγ and cancer-associated DM does not seem to be a chance relationship. There is a sound rationale, as this molecule has potent silencing activity based on repression of DNA transcription. Hypothetically, changes in the TIFIγ protein by cancer-related mutations, interactions among anti-TIFIγ antibodies, or other possible mechanisms could lead to poor functioning of the silencing activity, which would enable activation of certain DNA genes that are usually repressed. Although these theories have not been proven, this molecule is known to participate at the very onset of oncogenesis and is widely represented in a large number of tumours.

Therapeutic approach and prognosis of cancer-associated myositis

It is thought that in patients with cancer-associated myositis, treatment of cancer will lead to myositis resolution. However, this is not always the case. Occasionally, although a malignant tumour may be removed (e.g. localized colorectal cancer), the tumour antigens can act as triggers of the immune system and, even though the cancer is not present, the myositis may remain active. It is also sometimes difficult to determine whether treatment of the malignancy actually contributes to curing the myositis, because the immunosuppressive therapy used in some types of cancer, such as the R-CHOP (cyclophosphamide, doxorubicin, vincristine, and prednisolone-rituximab) scheme for patients with lymphoproliferative diseases, helps to modify the myositis as well due to strong immunosuppressive effects.

Data from several studies indicate that the presence of cancer in patients with myositis is a poor prognostic sign, also true in our experience. In these patients, the response of the malignancy to the current antineoplastic therapies is usually the factor that determines overall prognosis, not the complications related to the associated myositis. Nevertheless, studies focused on determining whether an earlier diagnosis of cancer will improve the overall prognosis are lacking in myositis patients.

In patients with cancer-associated myositis, in addition to the specific antineo-plastic therapy (surgery, radiotherapy, or chemotherapy), we initially use a triple therapy for the myositis, which includes prednisone (1 mg/kg/day), ciclosporin (3–5 mg/kg/day), and intravenous immunoglobulin (0.4 g/kg/day), the latter for 5 days per month for 6 months. This myositis treatment is adjusted according to clinical response over time. Usually, the myositis symptoms are well controlled with this treatment, in non-neoplastic, as well as in paraneoplastic cases. Special care has to be taken to avoid possible interactions with the chemotherapy drugs being simultaneously used (e.g. excessive immunosuppression). Hence, close col-laboration with attending oncologists is recommended.

Specific clinical scenarios (clinical pearls)

Clinical scenario (1)

A 45-year-old woman had been recently diagnosed with DM. She experienced severe proximal muscle weakness, dysphagia, and arthritis. A characteristic helio-trope rash was observed on her upper eyelids and the Gottron's sign was evident on her knuckles. Muscle biopsy showed a perimysial inflammatory infiltrate and perifascicular atrophy. Treatment was initiated with prednisone (1 mg/kg/day) and ciclosporin (5 mg/kg/day), with a slight clinical improvement. The patient's medical history and thorough physical examination did not suggest presence of any type of neoplasm. Broad cancer screening focusing on gynaecological neo-plasms (gynaecological ultrasonography and mammography), and chest and abdominal CT scans showed no signs of cancer. One month later, the patient remained highly symptomatic and the possibility of cancer-associated myositis was raised. Whole-body PET/CT scanning demonstrated muscle uptake indica-tive of myositis, but no pathological uptake in other organs or internal struc-tures. Cancer-associated DM was therefore thought to be reasonably ruled out. Intravenous immunoglobulin therapy was added at the third month after diagnosis and the patient experienced a clear improvement, being able to rise from her chair without help. Seven months after the diagnosis, and while the patient was under treatment with prednisone, ciclosporin, and intravenous immunoglobulin with improvements in rash and muscle function, she was referred to our emergency department for acute hemiparesis. CT examination of the brain showed several lesions suggestive of metastases. At that time, the clinical examination detected a palpable mass in her right breast; fine needle aspiration cytology demonstrated an invasive ductal breast carcinoma. Anti-TIFIγ antibody was not determined because it had not yet been described.

Comment on clinical scenario (1)

This is an unpleasant, but not uncommon situation. In some DM patients, no matter how intensively you search for an occult malignancy, it remains undetected, at least with the use of morphological and functional tests. Although PET/CT appears a good option to detect occult malignancy, and more convenient for the patient than broad cancer screening (only a single examination), it may initially fail to reveal a neoplasm. This may be because the cancer is present only at the molecular level and is contained by the immune system, but still responsible for the clinical manifestations of dermatomyositis. At this stage the neoplasm would be too small to be radiologically or functionally detected, but when the immune system fails, full blown cancer dissemination with metastatic disease can appear. Analysis of certain biological parameters such as anti-TIFIγ antibodies may be useful for early cancer detection. Nevertheless, longitudinal studies focused on defining the role of these autoantibodies as predictors of cancer development are lacking in myositis patients.

Clinical scenario (2)

A 54-year-old woman had been seen for abdominal distension and was diagnosed with a high-grade serous ovarian carcinoma four months previously. Laparoscopy and debulking surgery were performed and the patient was treated with a monthly regimen of carboplatin-paclitaxel at a standard dose during the next 6 months. After administration of the last cycle, she began to experience proximal weakness, with difficulty getting up from a chair and even taking a shower. She was unable to comb her hair, and experienced choking when eating and drinking. A scaly, oedematous heliotrope rash appeared on her eyelids and erythematous skin changes were seen on her chest ('V' sign), and at the middle of her upper back ('shawl' sign), following a photosensitivity pattern. Gottron's sign was present on her fingers. Muscle biopsy confirmed the diagnosis of DM, which was considered paraneoplastic due to development four months after diagnosis of ovarian malignancy. Anti-TIFIγ antibody testing by blot assay was strongly positive.

The patient received treatment with prednisone 60mg/day, ciclosporin 150 mg/bid, and 30 g/day of intravenous immunoglobulin for 5 days with considerable improvement. After one month of treatment, muscle strength was normal and the skin abnormalities had disappeared. Treatment with paclitaxel was resumed. During the next two months, the ovarian cancer progressed, with extension to the liver and peritoneum, but DM remained quiescent. A new chemotherapy approach with pegylated liposomal doxorubicin was initiated and ciclosporin was temporarily withdrawn because of the described potential interactions.

Comment on clinical scenario (2)

This could be a typical case of paraneoplastic DM. The close temporal relationship reinforces the diagnosis of cancer-associated myositis, even though the clinical outcome did not seem to run in parallel with DM activity. Furthermore, and this is not unusual, it could be assumed that destruction of the malignant disease by drug therapy would be responsible for the release of tumour antigens, which in turn, would lead to the development of DM.

The outcome in this patient will likely be unfavourable because of the ovarian cancer, which will likely progress to death, although the DM seems well controlled with conventional therapy. Clinicians treating myositis have to bear in mind the considerable potential for drug interactions in oncologic patients receiving several antineoplastic schemes. Therefore, close and easy communication with the cancer specialists is highly recommended, so that these patients will have the best possible prognosis.

SUGGESTED READING

Bohan A, Peter JB. (1975). Polymyositis and dermatomyositis (second of two parts). N Engl J Med; **292**: 403–7.

Buchbinder R, Forbes A, Hall S, Dennett X, Giles G. (2001). Incidence of malignant disease in biopsy-proven inflammatory myopathy. A population-based cohort study. Ann Intern Med; **134**: 1087–95.

Dalakas MC. (2015). Inflammatory muscle diseases. N Engl J Med; **373**: 393–4.

Hill CL, Zhang Y, Sigurgeirsson B, et al. (2001). Frequency of specific cancer types in dermatomyositis and polymyositis: a population-based study. Lancet; **357**: 96–100.

Huang YL, Chen YJ, Lin MW, et al. (2009). Malignancies associated with dermatomyositis and polymyositis in Taiwan: a nationwide population-based study. Br J Dermatol; **161**: 854–60.

Labrador-Horrillo M, Martínez MA, Selva-O'Callaghan A, et al. (2012). Anti-TIF1γ antibodies (anti-p155) in adult patients with dermatomyositis: comparison of different diagnostic assays. Ann Rheum Dis; **71**: 993–6.

Levin MI, Mozaffar T, Al-Lozi MT, Pestronk A. (1998). Paraneoplastic necrotizing myopathy: clinical and pathological features. Neurology; **50**: 764–7.

Lu X, Yang H, Shu X, et al. (2014). Factors predicting malignancy in patients with polymyositis and dermatomyostis: a systematic review and meta-analysis. PLoS One; **9**: e94128.

Selva-O'Callaghan A, Grau JM, Gámez-Cenzano C, et al. (2010). Conventional cancer screening versus PET/CT in dermatomyositis/polymyositis. Am J Med; **123**: 558–62.

Selva-O'Callaghan A, Mijares-Boeckh-Behrens T, Solans-Laqué R, et al. (2002). The neural network as a predictor of cancer in patients with inflammatory myopathies. Arthritis Rheum; **46**: 2547–8.

Sigurgeirsson B, Lindelöf B, Edhag O, Allander E. (1992). Risk of cancer in patients with dermatomyositis or polymyositis. A population-based study. N Engl J Med; **326**: 363–7.

Tiniakou E, Mammen AL. (2015). Idiopathic inflammatory myopathies and malignancy: a comprehensive review. *Clin Rev Allergy Immunol*; **52**(1): 20–33.

Trallero-Araguás E, Rodrigo-Pendás JÁ, Selva-O'Callaghan A, et al. (2012). Usefulness of anti-p155 autoantibody for diagnosing cancer-associated dermatomyositis: a systematic review and meta-analysis. *Arthritis Rheum*; **64**: 523–32.

Troyanov Y, Targoff IN, Tremblay JL, Goulet JR, Raymond Y, Senécal JL. (2005). Novel classification of idiopathic inflammatory myopathies based on overlap syndrome features and autoantibodies: analysis of 100 French Canadian patients. *Medicine (Balt)*; **84**: 231–49.

Yang Z, Lin F, Qin B, Liang Y, Zhong R. (2015). Polymyositis/dermatomyositis and malignancy risk: a meta-analysis study. *J Rheumatol*; **42**: 282–91.

CHAPTER 9

Toxic myopathies

Arash H. Lahouti and Lisa Christopher-Stine

KEY POINTS

- Many drugs, including prescribed medications, may cause muscle damage, through diverse mechanisms
- Discontinuation of an offending drug often leads to resolution of myopathy
- Statins commonly cause myalgias or muscle cramps
- In rare instances, statins can trigger an autoimmune myopathy characterized by proximal muscle weakness, very high muscle enzyme levels, and the generation of anti-HMGCR autoantibodies
- Colchicine can cause vacuolar myopathy and a concomitant neuropathy
- Steroid myopathy is characterized by proximal muscle weakness initially involving the lower extremities and normal muscle enzyme levels.

Toxic myopathy symptoms range from myalgia and muscle cramps to severe weakness, bearing similarities to a number of other muscle conditions. Thus, when evaluating patients with muscle symptoms, an iatrogenic muscle problem should always be considered, so as to distinguish a toxic from any other myopathy early on, so as to prevent further muscle damage and to potentially reverse muscle injury by withdrawal of the toxic agent. Various commonly prescribed medications, as well as illicit drugs, may cause muscle damage. These substances may cause muscle injury through direct myotoxic effects, or indirectly through various mechanisms, such as electrolyte abnormalities and triggering or disinhibiting the immune system response.

Introduction

The clinical symptoms of toxic myopathies range from myalgia and muscle cramps to severe weakness, with resulting disability. Symptoms may appear within days of drug initiation, or manifest only months to years later. A number of other muscle conditions bear similarities to toxic myopathies, in clinical terms. Therefore, when evaluating patients with muscle symptoms, an iatrogenic muscle problem should always be considered. It is important to distinguish a toxic from another form of myopathy early on, so as to prevent further muscle damage. Additionally, most substance-induced muscle diseases settle once the offending agent is withdrawn.

Skeletal muscles are susceptible to injury via exposure to many substances. Many commonly prescribed medications, as well as illicit drugs including alcohol, may cause muscle damage (Table 9.1). These myotoxic substances cause muscle injury through direct toxic effects, or indirectly through various mechanisms such as electrolyte abnormalities (e.g. hypokalaemia), and by triggering or disinhibiting the immune system (e.g. statins). Certain substances may cause muscle damage through a combination of these effects. For example, alcohol exerts both direct toxic effects on muscle cells and indirect effects via perturbations of potassium homeostasis. Alcohol may also cause rhabdomyolysis secondary to the mechanical damage related to prolonged immobility or seizures. Myofibre toxic effects are also diverse. For example, vincristine interferes with microtubular function and intracellular trafficking of vacuoles, thereby leading to vacuolar accumulations. By contrast, anti-retroviral medications exert toxic effects on mitochondria, leading to muscle cell damage, while anti-neoplastic agents cause muscle

Table 9.1 Substances associated with myopathy, classified by their presumed pathogenesis	
Pathological features	Substance(s)
Mitochondrial toxicity	Nucleoside reverse-transcriptase inhibitors (zidovudine)
Microtubular dysfunction	Colchicine Vincristine
Type 2 fibre atrophy	Glucocorticoids
Rhabdomyolysis	Statins Imatinib Colchicine Alcohol and illicit drugs Venoms
Autoimmune myopathy	Ipilimumab Adalimumab Interferon alfa Imatinib Penicillamine
Necrotizing autoimmune myopathy	Statins
Lysosomal dysfunction	Amiodarone Antimalarial agents (chloroquine and hydroxychloroquine)

injury through other mechanisms. 'Radiation recall' is an inflammatory reaction occurring in previously irradiated areas, a reaction usually limited to the skin, but focal muscle involvement is described (Pentsova et al. 2012). Immune-related adverse effects (IRAE) are reported after treatment with novel chemotherapeutic agents. For example, ipilimumab, an anti-T-cell antigen 4 monoclonal antibody, exerts anti-neoplastic properties by improving immune surveillance at the expense of induced autoimmunity, including an autoimmune myopathy (Hunter et al. 2009).

Statin myopathy

Statins are generally well tolerated, although adverse muscle affects can lead to drug intolerance. The severity spectrum of statin-induced muscle symptoms is broad, ranging from troublesome, self-limited myalgias to severe and life-threatening rhabdomyolysis (Box 9.1). Up to 29% of statin treated patients experience muscle symptoms (Stroes et al. 2015), though very few experience the serious effects of necrotizing myopathy or rhabdomyolysis. The muscle adverse event report in randomized, placebo-controlled trials is remarkably lower than that seen in patient registries and clinical experience. This is because participants with comorbidities that would predispose them to a higher risk for muscle adverse events may have been excluded from those trials. Several factors are associated with increased risk of muscle symptoms, including female sex, older age, chronic kidney and liver disease, hypothyroidism, and concomitant administration of other myotoxic agents or medications that interfere with statin metabolism (Box 9.2). Available data suggest that both statin dosage and individual formulation may contribute to muscle symptoms. Statin formulation differences are at least partially explained by their pharmacokinetics and lipophilicity, and inter-drug interactions. Thus, hydrophilic statins appear less likely to enter myocytes, and so have less potential for myotoxicity. Atorvastatin, simvastatin,

---

Box 9.1 Spectrum of muscle-related adverse events induced by statins

- *Myalgia*: muscle symptoms (i.e. myalgia, muscle cramping) with a normal CK level
- *HyperCKaemia*: elevated CK levels without any muscle symptoms.
- *Myopathy*: muscle symptoms (myalgia, muscle cramping, and weakness) plus an elevated CK level
- *Statin-associated IMNM*: muscle symptoms (myalgia, muscle cramping, and weakness), plus obviously elevated CK levels (10–20 × ULN) plus anti-HMGCR autoantibody detection
- *Rhabdomyolysis*: severe muscle symptoms plus markedly elevated (>40 × ULN) CK level, plus myoglobinuria and/or acute kidney injury

> **Box 9.2** Factors predisposing for statin-induced muscle symptoms
>
> - Advanced age (older than 80 years)
> - Female sex
> - Asian ethnicity
> - Low body mass index
> - History of previous neuromuscular disease (e.g. necrotizing myopathy, McArdle disease, and malignant hyperthermia)
> - Hypothyroidism
> - Chronic kidney disease
> - Chronic liver disease
> - Organ transplant recipients
> - Severe trauma
> - Human immunodeficiency virus
> - Diabetes mellitus
> - Vitamin D deficiency
> - Drug interactions (concomitant use of certain drugs including gemfibrozil, macrolides, azole antifungal agents, protease inhibitors, and immunosuppressive drugs such as ciclosporin, and inhibitors of CYP450 isoenzymes can affect the metabolism of statins, increase circulating statin levels, and the risk for muscle adverse events)
> - Concurrent administration of other myotoxic agents (e.g. alcohol, illicit drugs, etc.)

and lovastatin appear associated with the highest risk for statin-induced muscle symptoms, whereas pravastatin and fluvastatin have the lowest risk (Parker et al. 2013; Bruckert et al. 2005). Also, meta-analyses suggest that higher statin doses are associated with a greater risk for adverse effects (Silva et al. 2013). The precise mechanisms of statin-associated muscle symptoms remain undetermined, but mitochondrial dysfunction, a change in muscle membrane excitability secondary to alterations in membrane cholesterol and impaired calcium signalling have all been suggested as potential mechanisms.

Statin-associated immune-mediated necrotizing myopathy

In rare instances, long-term exposure to statins is associated with drug-induced autoimmune myopathy, muscle histology showing prominent myonecrosis with a relative paucity of inflammation (thus 'necrotizing myopathy'), in combination with the detection of circulating autoantibodies to HMG-CoA reductase. Accordingly, the disease has been termed statin-induced immune-mediated necrotizing myopathy (IMNM). This may occur in two or three of every 100,000 statin treated patients, who usually present with proximal muscle weakness and very elevated muscle enzyme levels. Myalgia is reported by over 70% of IMNM patients and the median duration of statin therapy prior to muscle symptom onset is 38 months (Basharat et al. 2016). In most cases, creatine kinase (CK) levels are > 10 times the upper limit of normal. Difficulty swallowing and distal muscle weakness also occur. Other systemic manifestations, such as joint involvement, interstitial lung disease, and skin manifestations are rare. In contrast to patients with 'simple' statin-associated myalgias, IMNM patients continue to experience symptoms long after drug cessation. Electromyography (EMG) may show an irritable myopathy and muscle oedema is evident on magnetic resonance imaging. HMG-CoA reductase (HMGCR) is a key enzyme in cholesterol synthesis, and the pharmacologic target of statin medications. The detection of anti-HMGCR antibodies in a patient with proximal muscle weakness and elevated CK level strongly suggests an autoimmune myopathy, since this antibody is rarely present where statin-associated muscle symptoms are self-limiting (Mammen et al. 2012). Therefore, in statin-exposed patients with raised CK, but a negative anti-HMGCR antibody test, an alternative diagnoses should be considered, e.g. an idiopathic inflammatory myopathy.

In IMNM, light microscopy demonstrates myofibre necrosis and regeneration without prominent inflammatory cell infiltrates. There may be diffuse or focal upregulation of MHC-1 expression on myofibres. The association of anti-HMGCR myopathy with HLA-DRB1*11:01 suggests a genetic predisposition. This is a common allele in the population, so other genetic/environmental factors will probably interact to confer IMNM risk and HLA-DRB1*11:01 cannot be used for screening. The mechanism by which statins induce development of the anti-HMGCR antibody is currently unknown, though the antibody target resides alongside P450 on the inside of the endoplasmic reticulum, so functional interactions may be implicated. Further, a proportion of IMNM patients with anti-HMGCR antibodies report no prior history of statin exposure. Such patients tend to be younger and have more resistance to immunosuppressive therapy. It is suggested that statin induced overexpression of HMG-CoA reductase in genetically susceptible individuals may trigger production of the antibodies to create an autoimmune response (Longo and Mammen 2016).

Management of statin myopathies

Patients who develop statin-induced muscle symptoms should undergo a thorough medical evaluation, and all medications should be carefully reviewed to identify potential drug interactions that may cause or exacerbate muscle symptoms. Diagnostic testing may include CK levels and thyroid stimulating hormone. Urinary myoglobin may be tested if the clinical presentation suggests rhabdomyolysis. The National Lipid Association (NLA) guidelines recommend immediate statin cessation in patients presenting with severe and otherwise unexplained muscle weakness, and/or marked CK elevations (Bays et al. 2016). After statin cessation, symptoms, and CK level should be monitored closely. Anti-HMG-CoA reductase autoantibody testing is recommended only in patients with markedly elevated CK levels, which persists after drug cessation (Longo and Mammen 2016). In patients with persisting myopathy, further assessment by EMG and muscle biopsy are warranted.

Statin re-challenge

The issue of statin re-challenge is controversial. Increased cardiovascular risks should be weighed against the potential for re-inducing muscle symptoms. The NLA guideline recommends dose reduction, or switching to a different statin or administering the statin fewer than 7 days a week in patients previously statin intolerant. If CK levels on a statin were more than 10 times the ULN, an alternative statin may be use to rechallenge, with a lower dose. If rhabdomyolysis was suspected or proven, most experts would suggest the avoidance of statin rechallenge (Stroes et al. 2015; Bays et al. 2016). There is lack of data regarding rechallenge of statins in patients with statin-associated necrotizing myopathy; however, the authors' personal observational data suggests that statin-rechallenge should be avoided here, and alternative lipid-lowering strategies adopted.

Management of immune-mediated necrotizing myopathy associated with anti-HMGCR antibodies

Unlike other forms of statin-associated problems, discontinuation of statin therapy is not always sufficient to halt disease activity, so in some patients, use of immunosuppressive medications may be required. However, such patients should ideally be referred to an experienced neurologist or rheumatologist for further workup, especially as muscle biopsy and EMG will be required. Treatment of IMNM associated with anti-HMGCR antibodies, whether associated with statins or not, is largely borrowed from that of other autoimmune myopathies, and on clinical experience. Initial treatment with oral glucocorticoids may be appropriate. If initial symptoms are severe, additional immunosuppressive medications such as methotrexate, azathioprine, or mycophenolate mofetil may be considered. Intravenous immunoglobulin (IVIG) and rituximab are reserved for refractory cases. Preliminary data show that IVIG may be particularly effective and may be even considered as first-line therapy in patients with contraindications to corticosteroids (Mammen and Tiniakou 2015). Immunosuppressive medications may be tapered once patients recover their strength.

Myopathy associated with anti-retroviral medications

Nucleoside reverse-transcriptase inhibitors (NRTIs) are the oldest class of anti-retroviral medications, which inhibit viral reverse transcriptase and mitochondrial

DNA polymerase-gamma (mtDNA-γ). Inhibition of the latter causes depletion of mtDNA, resulting in mitochondrial toxicity. Alternatively, a recent study suggests that NRTIs may cause deletions in mtDNA (Payne et al. 2015). The resultant decrease in skeletal muscle mitochondrial gene expression causes impairment of oxidative phosphorylation, and an inadequate energy production. Further, leakage from the electron-transport chain causes an increase in reactive oxygen species production, with subsequent oxidative damage of contractile and other proteins.

Zidovudine (AZT) is the NRTI agent most commonly associated with myopathy. Clinical manifestations are indistinguishable from other forms of auto-immune myopathy and HIV-associated polymyositis. Patients typically present with an insidious onset proximal muscle weakness, myalgia, and wasting. Symptom onset may be within months to several years after zidovudine initiation. CK elevations are usually moderate and EMG reveals irritable myopathy. The absence of inflammatory cells and the presence of ragged red fibres on muscle biopsy are findings helpful in differentiating azidothymidine (AZT) myopathy from other HIV-associated myopathies. Muscle strength usually improves upon drug cessation and the muscle enzymes usually normalize within weeks. If not, further investigation are required.

Myopathy associated with antimalarial drugs

Chloroquine and hydroxychloroquine (HCQ) are antimalarial drugs commonly used to treat various rheumatic diseases. Occasionally, these agents cause muscle toxicity, by accumulating in lysosomes to raise intralysosomal Ph and thus inhibit lysosomal enzymes. This results in accumulation of phospholipids, glycogen, and amyloid B with a characteristic curvilinear body formation seen on electron microscopy. Patients with HCQ myopathy usually present with mild to moderate proximal weakness and a normal or slightly elevated CK. However, fatal cases of respiratory failure have been reported in association with HCQ myopathy. Light microscopy may reveal cytoplasmic vacuoles (Casado et al. 2006). Medication discontinuation is usually associated with a good recovery expected.

Steroid myopathy

Chronic use of glucocorticoid can induce steroid myopathy, enhancing catabolism, and inhibiting anabolism in skeletal muscles. Specifically, accelerated degradation of the myogenic regulatory factor MyoD after glucocorticoid exposure may reduce muscle development and regeneration. Patients with steroid myopathy commonly present with a gradual onset of symmetrical proximal muscle weakness, initially involving the lower extremities and with a normal CK level. Muscle biopsy reveals nonspecific histologic changes, such as: variation in fibre size, type 2 fibre atrophy, fatty replacement, and without inflammation (Askari et al. 1976). Sometimes the diagnosis is challenging, as in patients with underlying inflammatory myopathies who are being treated with glucocorticoids. Here, steroid tapering may be required to allow improvements of muscle strength, an observation suggesting the diagnosis of steroid myopathy.

Colchicine

Colchicine inhibits the polymerization of β-tubulin into microtubules, thereby inhibiting movement of intracellular granules. In skeletal muscle, this can lead to accumulation of autophagic vacuoles and development of myopathy. Individuals taking a second myotoxic agent, or those with impaired renal function or solid organ transplants may all be at risk. Affected individuals develop proximal muscle weakness and serum CK elevations, usually accompanied by distal sensory loss due to a concomitant peripheral neuropathy (Wilbur and Makowsky 2004). Muscle biopsies show accumulation of lysosomes (Figure 9.1) and electron microscopy reveals whorled membranous bodies. Muscle weakness usually resolves within 3–4 weeks of cessation of therapy, but the axonal neuropathy resolves more slowly.

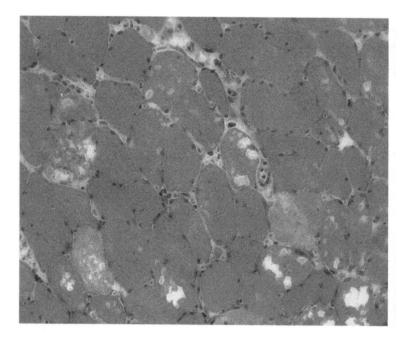

Figure 9.1 Colchicine myopathy. Frozen H&E shows vacuoles of varying size, situated both centrally, and right below the sarcolemma and often coalescing. Many vacuoles contain heterogeneous lysosomal material that stains positive on acid phosphatase.

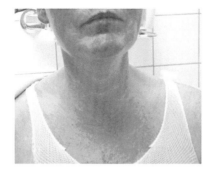

Figure 4.1 Characteristic skin feature in a patient with dermatomyositis: erythematous rash on the face, neck, and anterior chest (V sign) (a), Gottron's sign (A), palmar erythema (B), mechanic's hands (C), and/or mechanic's feet (D).

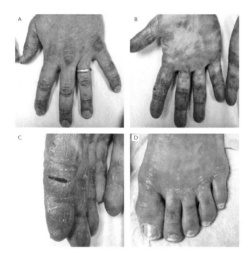

Figure 4.2 Characteristic skin feature in a patient with dermatomyositis: (A) red papules on the back of the finger joints (Gottron's sign), (B) palmar erythema, (C) mechanic's hands, and/or (D) mechanic's feet.

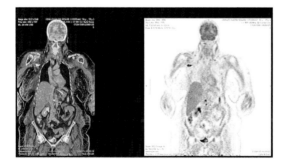

Figure 8.1 PET/CT images in a 67-year-old woman with refractory DM disclosed high uptake of lymphadenopathy at the upper and lower the diaphragm (SUVmax 23), suggestive of high-grade lymphoma, later confirmed by pathology.

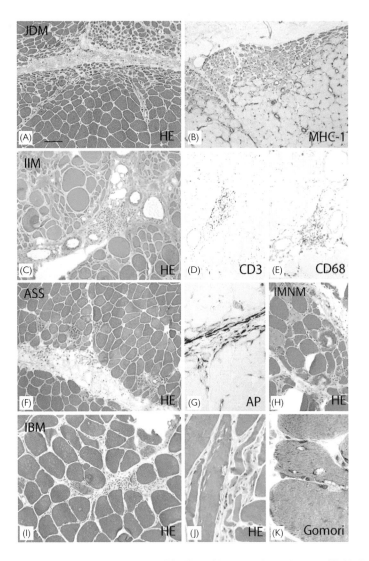

Figure 13.1 *Juvenile dermatomyositis* [(A) JDM, Haematoxylin and eosin; (B) H&E, major histocompatibility complex class I, MHC-1] showing perifascicular atrophy. *Non-specific* or *overlap myositis* (NSM/OM) in a patient with rheumatoid myositis [(C) H&E; (D) CD3; (E) CD68)] showing a perimysial perivascular cell infiltrate composed of CD3- positive lymphocytes and macrophages. *Antisynthetase syndrome* [ASS; (F) H&E; (G) alkaline phosphatase, AP] showing the presence of necrotic and regenerating fibres strongly clustered in perifascicular regions, and fragmentation of the perimysium staining intensely with AP. *Immune-mediated necrotizing myopathy (IMNM)*; (H) H&E, inclusion body myositis (I) H&E) showing an endomysial cell infiltrate invading a non-necrotic muscle fibre and rimmed vacuoles (J) H&E; (K) modified trichrome Gomori). Scale bar in A: (A–F) 80 mM; (G–J) 40 mM; (K) 20 mM.

REFERENCES

Askari A, Vignos PJ, Moskowitz RW. (1976). Steroid myopathy in connective tissue disease. *Am J Med*; **61**: 485–92.

Basharat P, Lahouti AH, Paik JJ, Albayda J, Pinal-Fernandez I, Bichile T, Lloyd TE, Danoff SK, Casciola-Rosen L, Mammen AL, Christopher-Stine L. (2016). Statin-Induced Anti-HMGCR-Associated Myopathy. *J Am Coll Cardiol*; **68**(2): 234–5.

Bays HE, Jones PH, Orringer CE, Brown WV, Jacobson TA. (2016). National Lipid Association Annual Summary of Clinical Lipidology 2016. *J Clin Lipidol*, **10**(Suppl. 1): S1–43.

Bruckert E, Hayem G, Dejager S, Yau C, Bégaud B. (2005). Mild to moderate muscular symptoms with high-dosage statin therapy in hyperlipidemic patients--the PRIMO study. *Cardiovasc Drugs Ther*; **19**: 403–14.

Casado E, Gratacós J, Tolosa C, et al. (2006). Antimalarial myopathy: an underdiagnosed complication? Prospective longitudinal study of 119 patients. *Ann Rheum Dis*; **65**: 385–90.

Hunter G, Voll C, Robinson CA. (2009). Autoimmune inflammatory myopathy after treatment with ipilimumab. *Canad J Neurol Sci*; **36**: 518–20.

Longo DL, Mammen AL. (2016). Statin-associated autoimmune myopathy. *N Engl J Med*; **374**: 664–9.

Mammen AL, Tiniakou E. (2015). Intravenous immune globulin for statin-triggered autoimmune myopathy. *N Engl J Med*; **373**: 1680–2.

Mammen AL, Pak K, Williams EK et al. (2012). Rarity of anti-3-hydroxy-3-methylglutaryl-coenzyme A reductase antibodies in statin users, including those with self-limited musculoskeletal side effects. *Arthritis Care Res (Hoboken)*; **64**: 269–72.

Payne BA, Gardner K, Blakely EL, et al. (2015). Clinical and pathological features of mitochondrial DNA deletion disease following antiretroviral treatment. *J Am Med Assoc Neurol*; **72**: 603–5.

Parker BA, Capizzi JA, Grimaldi AS, et al. (2013). Effect of statins on skeletal muscle function. *Circulation*; **127**: 96–103.

Pentsova E et al. (2012). Gemcitabine induced myositis in patients with pancreatic cancer: case reports and topic review. *J Neurooncol*, **106**, 15–21.

Silva M et al. (2007). Meta-analysis of drug-induced adverse events associated with intensive-dose statin therapy. *Clin Ther*, **29**, 253–60.

Stroes ES et al. (2015). Statin-associated muscle symptoms: impact on statin therapy-European Atherosclerosis Society Consensus Panel Statement on Assessment, Aetiology and Management. *Eur Heart J*; **36**: 1012–22.

Wilbur K, Makowsky M. (2004). Colchicine myotoxicity: case reports and literature review. *Pharmacotherapy*; **24**: 1784–92.

CHAPTER 10

Juvenile myositis

Christina Boros, K. Nistala, and L.R. Wedderburn

KEY POINTS

- Key differences exist between adult and paediatric inflammatory myopathies
- Use of recently described clinical and serological classification criteria should improve our ability to perform standardized research in these conditions
- New treatment options will likely improve long term outcomes. The development of a robust evidence-base for their use requires international collaborative studies.

Introduction

The idiopathic inflammatory myopathies (IIM) occur rarely in childhood, with the most common form, juvenile dermatomyositis (JDM), having an incidence of only 3–4 per million children per year. Significant morbidity and mortality still exist in these disorders, in particular in those with severe skin involvement such as calcinosis or ulceration, as well as those with major organ involvement, such as GI tract or interstitial lung disease (ILD). Therefore, early recognition of JDM and its complications, and institution of appropriate management are extremely important.

Classification

The original classification criteria for JDM published by Bohan and Peter in 1975 did not allow for the fact that childhood IIM represent a heterogeneous disease spectrum. In addition, although electromyography (EMG) and/or muscle biopsy may be necessary to provide correct classification, both are often considered too invasive in paediatric cases. There is a move towards muscle magnetic resonance imaging replacing these investigations, but this may also still require general anaesthesia, as the commonest age at diagnosis is 6–7 years.

Clinical classification describes subgroups which are the same as in adults, but with different relative frequencies and prognoses, and sometimes also with different features at presentation. JDM is the commonest juvenile IIM, occurring in approximately 85% of cases with overlap myositis in 9–10% of cases, juvenile polymyositis in 4–5%, amyopathic/hypomyopathic variants in 1% and other variants in < 1% of cases (Tansley et al. 2013).

However, because existing criteria are inadequate for standardized clinical research, an international multidisciplinary collaboration, the International Myositis Classification Criteria Project (IMCCP), was established to develop new classification criteria for both Juvenile and Adult IIM.

Much recent research has focused on serological classification in childhood IIM, and its relationship with clinical phenotype. It has now been determined that approximately 70% of children have a myositis-specific autoantibodies (MSA). Several MSA are found in adults and children, but their prevalence differs considerably, and depending on age at onset. Some MSA provide clear prognostic value in JDM, but again the clinical features associated with specific MSA vary in frequency between adults and children. For example, anti-p155/140 (TIF1γ) is much commoner in JDM than in adult dermatomyositis (DM; 32% vs 10%), whereas anti-synthetase Abs are considerably more common in adult DM. However, whether serological subgroups will be distinct enough to provide a robust classification of childhood IIM remains to be determined.

Differences between adult and paediatric disease

Clinical

IIM are less common in childhood than in adults; rash in childhood IIM can occur anywhere on the body and is more likely to be ulcerative than in adults. Polymyositis and amyopathic/hypomyopathic disease are less common in childhood and paediatric disease, but appears to have better treatment response. Creatine kinase is less consistently raised in juvenile myositis than in adult IIM so the testing of other muscle enzymes is recommended (Enders et al. 2017).

ILD is more common in adults, and is associated with poorer prognosis than when occurring in childhood: 3.5% of children vs 49% of adults have lung damage at long-term follow-up. However, some 40% of IIM children have asymptomatic pulmonary function test abnormalities (Tansley et al. 2013). Conversely, calcinosis is more common in childhood disease, and is typically a later sign associated with delayed diagnosis, a chronic course, and inadequate treatment. Other major organ vasculopathy is also more common in childhood (Tansley et al. 2013).

DM is considered to be a paraneoplastic syndrome in adults and is associated with triple the risk of all types of cancer reported compared with the general population. However, while there have been individual case reports of malignancy in paediatric IIM, there is no clear association. The presence of anti- TIF1γ Ab appears not to be associated with cancer in childhood, unlike the frequent association with malignancy in adults

Serological

In addition to the differences seen in TIF1γ Ab associations, children with anti-synthetases are more likely to have overlap myositis (versus polymyositis in adults), to present with falls and muscle atrophy, and be less likely to have ILD, mechanics' hands, and Raynaud's phenomenon. Children with anti-Mi-2 are more likely to exhibit V- or shawl-sign rashes, and have more cuticular overgrowth, whereas adults have a higher incidence of carpal tunnel syndrome (Rider et al. 2013).

Anti-NXP2 is found in 11–23% of children with myositis, but in only 1.6% of adult IIM patients. In JDM, anti-NXP2 antibody is strongly associated with calcinosis development, and a more severe disease course, with persistent disease activity and poor functional status (Tansley et al. 2013; Rider et al. 2013). The anti-MDA 5 antibody is associated with relatively mild muscle disease, but more rash and a higher risk of ILD in children (Tansley et al. 2014).

Pathophysiological

Although disease pathogenesis and genetic susceptibility are similar in adult and paediatric disease, childhood myositis is associated with more prevalent vasculopathy, increased neovascularization of capillaries, a greater degree of C5b–9 complement deposition in affected muscles, increased major histocompatibility complex (MHC) class I up-regulation on myofibres and increased type I IFN signature in comparison to adult disease (Robinson and Reed 2011). An internationally agreed standardized method to assess features and severity on muscle biopsy has enabled a more robust comparison of the pathophysiology between cases (Varsani et al. 2015) and, interestingly, the data scored on biopsy has recently been shown to be predictive of outcome in a study of 101 biopsies (Deakin et al. 2016).

Outcomes

Previous studies have suggested that only one third of children with IIM have a chronic disease course, but more recent evidence seems to contradict this. Sanner et al., reported reduced quality of life and educational, and employment opportunities, as well as impaired cardiac and lung functions, higher rates of disease activity (51%), and end organ damage (90%) in comparison with healthy controls in a cohort of 60 Norwegian patients studied cross-sectionally at a median of 16.8 years post-JDM diagnosis (Sanner et al. 2010). Mathiesen et al. have also published similar findings (60% with end organ damage) in a Danish cohort of 57 JDM patients with a median follow-up of 13.9 years.

The largest outcome study to date (Ravelli et al. 2010), which included 490 JDM children from 27 European and South American centres seen 2–25 years after diagnosis, again using cross-sectional clinical assessment and retrospective chart review, found that most participants reported good Health Related Quality of Life (HRQoL) with few exhibiting severe muscle weakness or physical disability, but nonetheless, 40–60% had persistently active disease.

Mortality rates, though overall much reduced with modern treatment, are increased in JDM for those with overlap myositis and anti-synthetase Abs. A standardized mortality ratio (SMR) in JDM of 2.64 was reported in a US paediatric rheumatic disease registry including 662 patients with JDM (five deaths in

50,000 patients from 60 centres, mean follow-up 7.9 years) and, in a US juvenile myositis cohort of 405 patients with a mean follow-up of 4.4 years, a SMR of 14.4 (17 deaths) was reported for the entire cohort and of 8.3 (eight deaths) for JDM (Hashkes et al. 2010; Huber et al. 2014).

Treatment of juvenile dermatomyositis

The aim of JDM treatment is to control muscle and skin inflammation using immunosuppressive drugs, and physical therapy to restore normal muscle function. Corticosteroids have been the mainstay of treatment since the 1950s, and have been instrumental in reducing mortality in juvenile and adult IIM. However, several questions remain; the first, whether steroid treatment alone is sufficient? This was addressed in a recent randomized controlled trial led by the Paediatric Rheumatology International Trials Organisation (PRINTO) group (Ruperto et al. 2016). The results suggest that adding methotrexate or ciclosporin achieves better disease control compared with steroids alone, and of the two disease modifying anti-rheumatic drugs (DMARDS), methotrexate has a better side effect profile. Unfortunately, the trial did not address which is the best steroid dose, route of administration or weaning strategy. Paediatric rheumatologists from the USA and Europe have drawn up consensus based recommendations on therapy (Huber et al. 2012). For patients with moderately severe disease, both groups recommend initial therapy with high dose intravenous methylprednisolone followed by 1–2 mg/kg oral prednisone, which is then weaned over 9–12 months; a regime that unfortunately leads to significant steroid toxicity. For patients with severe disease at presentation [Childhood Myositis Assessment Scale (CMAS) <15, Manual Muscle Testing-8 (MMT8) <30, nasopharyngeal involvement, cutaneous ulceration or other organ involvement] there was limited consensus. At the authors' institution patients are treated with 500 mg/m^2 IV cyclophosphamide at 2–4 weekly intervals for 5–7 doses, followed by maintenance therapy with methotrexate (Riley et al. 2004).

Active monitoring of disease activity using validated score tools is important in all patients, and those failing to respond should be considered for additional therapy, such as intravenous immunoglobulin (IVIG), cyclophosphamide, biologic agents, or a change of DMARD to mycophenolate mofetil (Dagher et al. 2012). A US-based study of adults and children tested the efficacy of rituximab, but failed to meet its primary trial end point. Nevertheless, >70% of patients with disease resistant to first line therapy still met the ACR definition of improvement, with better responses in seropositive patients (Aggarwal et al. 2014). Anti-TNFα therapies have been reported to be effective in the treatment of calcinosis, and skin disease resistant to IVIG and methotrexate. There have been concerns in the adult literature with a case series of 17 RA patients who developed new onset DM and PM following anti-TNFα therapy, though this signal has not been seen in juvenile arthritis (Brunasso et al. 2014).

Historically, the management of calcinosis has divided experts, with many suggesting that calcinosis represents disease damage. At a recent EU funded initiative of JDM experts (Single Hub and Access point Paediatric Rheumatology, SHARE) there was consensus that new or worsening calcinosis may represent active skin inflammation, and escalation of therapy should be considered (Enders et al. 2017).

Withdrawal of therapy

Most centres advocate continuing methotrexate for a year after achieving clinically inactive disease off steroids (Lazarevic et al. 2013; Almeida et al. 2015). Unlike in adult DM, once in remission, children are unlikely to relapse after stopping treatment. There are several emerging biomarkers that may detect subclinical inflammation in JDM, and these may further reduce the risk of relapse (Nistala et al. 2013).

Future treatment directions

Reducing steroid toxicity and managing treatment resistant skin disease currently represent major challenges facing clinicians treating JDM. New therapeutic approaches targeting the interferon pathway offer promise. Blockade of type I interferons has shown some benefit in adult myositis patients, but there are currently few published data. Drugs which block pathways downstream of type I interferons, such as Janus Kinase (JAK) inhibitors, may attenuate many of the inflammatory pathways involved in DM. In the early onset genetic condition chronic atypical neutrophilic dermatosis with lipodystrophy and elevated temperature (CANDLE), caused by mutations in the proteasome subunits, which shares some features with JDM and is known to involve over-production of interferon IFN, these drugs have shown benefit in initial studies. If these new treatments achieve better disease control, then the natural ability of childhood muscle to undergo repair and regeneration offers a better outlook for children with this rare, but serious disorder.

Transition

While there are no studies specific for transition in childhood inflammatory myopathies, there is a growing literature regarding transition medicine in paediatric rheumatology, which has led the way in providing the evidence base on which current models of care are being developed for all paediatric patients. The skills young people need to acquire during this process include self-management, health literacy, and the ability to comply with medications and management plans. The acquisition of these skills is dependent upon cognitive developmental level, rather than age. Therefore, as much as possible, transition should be an individualized process.

An important concept in transition is that many biological and developmental tasks are faced even by healthy adolescents, which include significant frontal lobe synaptic pruning and the associated, well-recognized behaviour changes. In adolescents with chronic disease, these changes can impact upon the prevalence of health-related risk behaviours, which include smoking, alcohol, and recreational drug use, unsafe sexual practices, as well as non-compliance with medication and other therapies. Therefore health professionals involved in transition processing should be appropriately trained to elicit and discuss such behaviours, and be able to work with young people to provide appropriate management plans.

The concept of transition should be discussed early, often as young 11–12 years, if developmentally appropriate. Adolescents with IIM and other rheumatologic disorders often require multidisciplinary and multispecialty care, so inclusion of interested and enthusiastic adult, as well as paediatric practitioners in the transition team is important. In addition, young people prefer and need the opportunity to meet their adult healthcare providers in outpatient clinics sometimes without parents being present, prior to transition.

Parents' needs during this process should also be considered, as they can assist their child's acquisition of appropriate skills. In addition, transition will often cause parental anxiety, as it involves a major shift in care paradigm for them as well as their child.

Also of great importance is the provision of a comprehensive health record to all adult practitioners, and held by the adolescent themselves. Tracking mechanisms should be put in place to ensure that adolescents and young people do not become lost to follow-up, and thus continuity of care.

There is no single model of care proven to be better than others, but successful models include those including employment of a jointly–funded co-ordinator to address transitional care across institutions, development of clinics in which adolescents can see both their paediatric and adult teams at the same institution and development of young adult rheumatology services for those 16–25 years in age (Tattersall and McDonagh 2010).

Future directions

As childhood IIM are so rare it is vital that International collaborations allow maximal use of data and knowledge from all available cases. An International group of experts has thus agreed to develop a minimal dataset for use in clinical and research settings, allowing all childhood IIM cases to be compared and shared in a robust way. The proposed data set will be aligned with other on-going data collections and registries, such as the JDM component of an International Registry for IIM, i.e. Euromyositis. These efforts, combined with European initiatives to propose best practice standards for children and young people with JDM (SHARE) should allow all children to receive optimal pathways in this complex and difficult disease.

REFERENCES

Aggarwal R Bandos A, Reed AM, et al. (2014). Predictors of clinical improvement in rituximab-treated refractory adult and juvenile dermatomyositis and adult polymyositis. *Arthritis Rheumatol (Hoboken)*; **66**: 740–9.

CHAPTER 10

Almeida B, Campanilho-Marques R, Arnold K, et al. (2015). Analysis of Published Criteria for Clinically Inactive Disease in a Large Juvenile Dermatomyositis Cohort Shows That Skin Disease Is Underestimated. *Arthritis Rheumatol (Hoboken)*; **67**: 2495–502.

Brunasso AM, Aberer W, Massone C. (2014). New onset of dermatomyositis/polymyositis during anti-TNF-alpha therapies: a systematic literature review. *ScientificWorldJournal*; **2014**: 179180.

Dagher R, Desjonquères M, Duquesne A, et al. (2012). Mycophenolate mofetil in juvenile dermatomyositis: a case series. *Rheumatol Int*; **32**: 711–16.

Deakin CT, Yasin SA, Simou S, et al. (2016). Muscle biopsy in combination with myositis-specific autoantibodies aids prediction of outcomes in juvenile dermatomyositis. *Arthritis Rheumatol (Hoboken)*; **68**: 2806–16.

Enders FB, Bader-Meunier B, Baildam E, et al. (2017). Consensus based recommendations for the management of juvenile dermatomyositis. *Ann Rheum Dis*; **76**: 329–40.

Hashkes PJ, Wright BM, Lauer MS, et al. (2010). Mortality outcomes in pediatric rheumatology in the US. *Arthritis Rheum*; **62**: 599–608.

Huber AM, Mamyrova G, Lachenbruch PA, et al. (2014). Early illness features associated with mortality in the juvenile idiopathic inflammatory myopathies. *Arthritis Care Res*; **66**: 732–40.

Huber AM, Robinson AB, Reed AM, et al. (2012). Consensus treatments for moderate juvenile dermatomyositis: beyond the first two months. Results of the second Childhood Arthritis and Rheumatology Research Alliance consensus conference. *Arthritis Care Res*; **64**: 546–53.

Larazevic D, Pistorio A, Palmisani E et al. (2013). The PRINTO criteria for clinically inactive disease in juvenile Dermatomyositis. *Ann Rheum Dis*; **72**: 686–93.

Nistala K, Varsani H, Wittowski H, et al. (2013). Myeloid related protein induces muscle derived inflammatory mediators in juvenile dermatomyositis. *Arthritis Res Ther*; **15**: R131.

Ravelli A, Trail L, Ferrari C, et al. (2010). Long-term outcome and prognostic factors of juvenile dermatomyositis: a multinational, multicenter study of 490 patients. *Arthritis Care Res*; **62**: 63–72.

Rider LG, Shah M, Mamyrova G, et al. (2013). The myositis autoantibody phenotypes of the juvenile idiopathic inflammatory myopathies. *Medicine*; **92**: 223–43.

Riley P, Maillard SM, Wedderburn LR, et al. (2004). Intravenous cyclophosphamide pulse therapy in juvenile dermatomyositis. A review of efficacy and safety. *Rheumatol (Oxf)*; **43**: 491–6.

Robinson AB, Reed AM. (2011). Clinical features, pathogenesis and treatment of juvenile and adult dermatomyositis. *Nature Rev Rheumatol*; **7**: 664–75.

Ruperto N, Pistorio A, Oliveira S, et al. (2016). Prednisone versus prednisone plus ciclosporin versus prednisone plus methotrexate in new-onset juvenile dermatomyositis: a randomised trial. *Lancet*; **387**: 671–8.

Sanner H, Kirkhus E, Merckoll E, et al. (2010). Long-term muscular outcome and predisposing and prognostic factors in juvenile dermatomyositis: a case-control study. *Arthritis Care Res*; **62**: 1103–11.

Tansley SL, Betteridge ZE, Gunawardena H, et al. (2014). Anti-MDA5 autoantibodies in juvenile dermatomyositis identify a distinct clinical phenotype: a prospective cohort study. *Arthritis Res Ther*; **16**: R138.

Tansley SL, McHugh NJ, Wedderburn LR (2013). Adult and juvenile dermatomyositis: are the distinct clinical features explained by our current understanding of serological subgroups and pathogenic mechanisms? *Arthritis Res Ther*; **15**: 211.

Tattersall R, McDonagh JE. (2010). Transition: a rheumatology perspective. *Br J Hosp Med*; **71**: 315–19.

Varsani H, Charman SC, Li CK, et al. (2015). Validation of a score tool for measurement of histological severity in juvenile dermatomyositis and association with clinical severity of disease. *Ann Rheum Dis*; **74**: 204–10.

CHAPTER 11

Inclusion body myositis

Pedro M. Machado

KEY POINTS

- In inclusion body myositis (IBM), significant delays occur between symptom onset and diagnosis. Asymmetric finger flexor and knee extensor weakness are characteristic clinical features

- Diagnostic muscle biopsy features are highly specific in combination, but lack sensitivity. Current evidence favours p62 as the most discriminatory and reliable immuno-staining technique

- New European Neuromuscular Centre (ENMC) diagnostic criteria will facilitate earlier patient enrolment in future clinical trials

- Magnetic resonance imaging (MRI) has potential utility as an outcome measure for future IBM clinical trials

- Auto-antibodies against cytosolic 5'-nucleotidase 1A may have diagnostic utility in IBM

- The pathogenesis of IBM remains elusive. Evidence accumulates for roles for autoimmunity, mitochondrial dysfunction, protein dyshomeostasis, altered nucleic acid metabolism, and myonuclear degeneration

- No evidence supports the prolonged use of immunosuppressive agents in IBM, but individual cases with high levels of inflammation may gain short term benefit from such medication

- Supportive management by muscle experts is recommended and individualized exercise programmes may benefit some patients. Targeting protein dyshomeostasis may be a promising therapeutic approach in IBM.

Introduction

Inclusion body myositis (IBM) is an acquired muscle disease with a male predominance, and rarely affects individuals below the age of 45 years. A recent Norwegian study estimated an IBM prevalence of 33/million (compared with 87/million for PM/DM combined). The rarity of IBM, the lack of patient and clinical awareness, and diagnostic difficulties contribute to significant delays between symptom onset and diagnosis, the average delay being some 5 years.

Clinical features, natural history, and outcome measures

Historically, IBM was regarded as an idiopathic inflammatory myopathy (IIM), grouped with polymyositis (PM), dermatomyositis (DM), and other immune-mediated myopathies. However, IBM clearly differs from these other IIM and is characterized by a lack of treatment response to immunosuppressant medications. It also exhibits inflammatory and degenerative features histologically, a characteristic clinical phenotype clearly different to PM/DM, with (often asymmetric) weakness of the knee extensors (manifesting early on as falls) and finger flexors (manifesting as grip impairment). It has a relentless and usually slow progression that causes severe disability and loss of quality of life. Dysphagia can be an early feature, though usually presenting late and representing a risk factor for aspiration-associated deaths. Pharyngeal and oesophageal dysfunction may also contribute to malnutrition. Ankle dorsiflexion and facial weakness may also be seen at an early stage. There is no consistent association with malignancy or extra-articular manifestations. Most reports show no decrease in life expectancy in IBM, although a recent Norwegian study did demonstrate a standardized mortality rate of 1.7 in IBM, compared with 2.6 in DM and 2.4 in PM.

IBM is often initially misdiagnosed as PM. The recognition of the typical weakness of finger flexors and knee extensors, the late onset of the disease (i.e. > 45–50 years), the slow disease progression, and the demonstration of supportive biopsy findings are key to making an accurate diagnosis. Repeated muscle biopsies may thus be required. Inconclusive results are often found in patients with an initial PM diagnosis, but which proves refractory to immunosuppressive treatment. Such patients, or those developing atypical clinical features, should always have their diagnosis reconsidered and biopsy repeated if necessary. Other muscle diseases with potential for inflammatory features should be borne in mind in the differential diagnosis, as discussed in earlier chapters.

IBM disease progression is variable and no robust outcome predictors are available. Male gender, older age at onset, and use of immunosuppressive agents (paradoxically) are all factors predictive of progression towards walking handicap (though not predictive of progression towards wheelchair use). Mean percentage decline in muscle strength is reported as 3.1–9.1% per year, with considerable variability at the individual level. After 10 years, most patients need some type of walking aid and after 15 years most require wheelchairs.

Appropriate outcome measures for IBM clinical trials are lacking. Data suggest that quantitative quadriceps muscle testing and the IBM functional rating scale may be sensitive tools to monitor disease progression. The IBM functional assessment (sIFA) scale is another disease-specific physical function scale. In the largest, randomized, double blind, placebo-controlled IBM trial (RDBPCT) to date (NCT01925209), assessment of mobility via a 6-min walk distance test (6MWD) was the primary outcome measure. Swallowing function can be assessed using video-fluoroscopy and the swallowing quality of life survey (SWAL-QOL). Recently real time MRI has been proposed to assess dysphagia in IBM. Further research is needed to determine the longitudinal relationship between changes in these outcome measures, as well as their discriminatory capacity and responsiveness.

Investigations

Laboratory abnormalities

Muscle enzymes are typically elevated in IBM, with CK levels generally being <10–12 times normal. Markers of systemic inflammation, such as acute phase reactant elevations and chronic anaemia, are usually absent.

Electromyography usually reveals a myopathic pattern with increased insertional activity, fibrillations, and polyphasic potentials, findings that are not IBM specific. A mixed pattern of myopathic and neurogenic changes is also common in IBM. Nerve conduction studies are usually normal.

Autoantibodies against cytosolic 5'-nucleotidase 1A (cN1A) represent a new serological biomarker for IBM, and potentially useful in the differential diagnosis of recent onset myopathies/myositis. However, no consensus exists regarding the most appropriate method for detecting anti-cN1A auto-antibodies. Also, anti-cN-1A auto-antibodies are often also found in patients with Sjögren's syndrome and systemic lupus erythematosus.

Histopathological findings

In addition to inflammatory changes, IBM muscle histology (Figure 11.1) also reveals a range of other pathological features, including: variation in fibre size, rounded, and angulated atrophic fibres, increased numbers of internalized nuclei, mitochondrial changes including cytochrome c oxidase (COX)-negativity, succinate dehydrogenase (SDH)-positive fibres, ragged red fibres, and increased endomysial connective tissue.

Historically, diagnostic criteria for IBM depended heavily on the demonstration of characteristic pathological findings, the Griggs et al. criteria being the first adopted for IBM. These dictate that a diagnosis of definite IBM can be made solely by the presence of: an auto-aggressive inflammatory myopathy with invasion of morphologically normal fibres, presence of rimmed vacuoles (irregular vacuoles within a muscle fibre surrounded by, or containing basophilic granular material with haematoxylin and eosin staining or staining red with Gomori trichrome), and either amyloid or 15–18 nm tubulofilamentous inclusions visualized by electron microscopy (EM). However, these findings are not always present in initial biopsies, and are also sometimes found in isolation in other myopathies. The subsequent recognition of characteristic IBM clinical features has revealed that histological features thought diagnostic in IBM may in fact be absent in patients with clinically typical IBM. One study found that >40% of IBM patients diagnosed clinically lacked diagnostic pathological features at presentation. The limited sensitivity of the pathological features included in the Griggs et al. criteria is likely because they associate with advanced disease only.

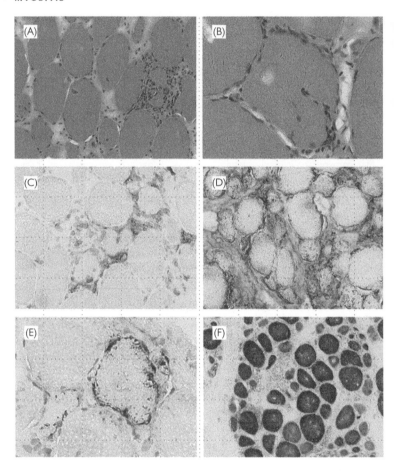

Figure 11.1 Muscle biopsy from IBM patient showing endomysial inflammation (A, ×20), partial invasion, and a rimmed vacuole (B, ×40), infiltration by CD8+ T-cells (C, ×20), MHC Class I up-regulation (D, ×20), p62 positive fibres (E, ×40), and COX-negative SDH-positive fibres (F, ×10). MHC, major histocompatibility complex; COX, cytochrome c oxidase; SDH, succinate dehydrogenase.

Immunohistochemical staining techniques have clarified the composition of inflammatory infiltrates in IBM, revealed widespread sarcolemma and sarcoplasmic upregulation of MHC class I (MHC-I) and identified pathological accumulations of abnormal proteins within IBM myofibres. The proteins described include many commonly associated with neurodegenerative diseases: β-amyloid, phosphorylated tau, and ubiquitin; myofibrillar myopathy associated proteins: myotilin and αB-crystallin; and newer neurodegenerative markers: p62 and TDP-43. These findings have not been consistently reproduced. The following pattern of p62 immunoreactivity has been proposed as being highly characteristic of IBM: strongly stained, discreet, and clearly delineated, round or angular aggregates, variable in number and size within a muscle fibre, but rarely filling it and predominantly located in the subsarcolemma, but also perinuclear and adjacent to vacuoles.

MRI assessment

Muscle MRI is recognized as useful for diagnosis of inherited and acquired muscle diseases. In IBM patients, muscle signal hyperintensity on T1-weighted sequences, due to intramuscular fat accumulation, and signal hyperintensity on T2-weighted sequences with fat suppression (e.g. STIR) sequences, due to muscle oedema, are seen (Figure 11.2). Selective muscle involvement patterns are reported. Matching the clinical presentation, there is preferential forearm intramuscular fat accumulation within flexor digitorum profundus while, in the thigh, quadriceps femoris is preferentially affected. STIR hyperintensity reflecting active muscle inflammation is often seen, but in a smaller number of muscles than those affected by fat accumulation. Although this is a typical pattern of involvement, the diagnostic sensitivity and specificity of MRI has not been systematically assessed in IBM, and MRI appearances are not currently included in IBM diagnostic criteria.

In addition to its diagnostic role, MRI also shows promise as a tool for monitoring disease progression, as is can quantify intramuscular fat accumulation and water content. In IBM, MRI has thus been shown to:

- Monitor intramuscular fat accumulation with high responsiveness.
- Correlate well with functional measures.
- Detect muscle water changes preceding marked intramuscular fat accumulation.

These results suggest that MRI biomarkers might prove valuable in future clinical trials. Unlike strength testing, MRI is independent of volition, so may provide a more reliable measure of disease progression than manual muscle testing.

Diagnostic criteria

The earliest diagnostic criteria, of Griggs et al., were heavily weighted towards pathological features, while later criteria give increased importance to clinical features. The 2011 ENMC diagnostic criteria, the latest IBM diagnostic criteria, build on the previously published Medical Research Council (MRC) criteria. In the presence of the appropriate clinical phenotype, the ENMC criteria allow more flexibility regarding the presence of typical histopathological features. Patients can be

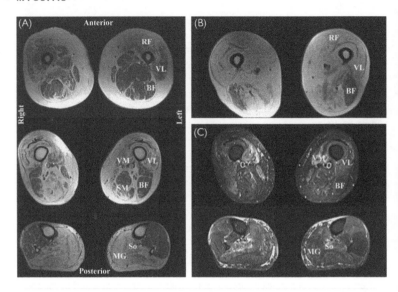

Figure 11.2 Typical MRI appearances in an IBM patient. (A) Axial T1-weighted images of the mid-thigh (top), distal thigh (middle), and mid-calf (bottom). This shows intramuscular fat accumulation, evident as hyperintensity, most notably within quadriceps (RF, rectus femoris; VL, vastus lateralis; VM, vastus medialis) especially in the distal thigh. Hamstring involvement is asymmetric with semimembranosus (SM) relatively spared on the left. In the calf the medial gastrocnemius (MG) is completely replaced by fat, with soleus (So) also severely affected. (B) Axial T1-weighted image at mid-thigh of the same patient 6 years later shows significant progression of intramuscular fat accumulation, with only biceps femoris (BF) relatively unaffected. (C) Axial STIR images at distal thigh (top) and mid-calf (calf) in the same patient at baseline. Acute muscle inflammation is evident as hyperintensity, most markedly in vastus medialis and soleus.

divided into three categories: 'clinicopathologically defined IBM', 'clinically defined IBM', and 'probable IBM' (Table 11.1).

Pathogenesis

Multiple hypotheses regarding IBM pathogenesis are proposed (Figure 11.3). Environmental factors (e.g. viral infection), ageing, genetic susceptibility, autoimmunity, accumulation of toxic proteins, myonuclear degeneration, endoplasmic reticulum stress, impairment of autophagy, disruption of the ubiquitin-proteasome system, and myostatin signalling, mitochondrial dysfunction and alterations of nucleic metabolism all have been proposed as contributing to IBM pathogenesis.

Table 11.1 European Neuromuscular Centre Inclusion Body Myositis research diagnostic criteria 2011

Diagnostic sub-group	Clinicopathologically defined IBM	Clinically defined IBM	Probable IBM
Clinical features			
Duration of weakness > 12 months	X	X	X
Age at onset > 45 years	X	X	X
Creatine kinase ≤ 15× ULN	X	X	X
FF weakness > SA weakness **and/or** KE weakness ≥ HF weakness	X	–	–
FF weakness > SA weakness **and** KE weakness ≥ HF weakness	–	X	–
FF weakness > SA weakness **or** KE weakness ≥ HF weakness	–	–	X
Pathological features			
Endomysial inflammatory infiltrate	X	≥1, but not all of the four pathological features	≥1, but not all of the four pathological features
Rimmed vacuoles	X		
Protein accumulation* or 15–18nm filaments	X		
Up-regulation of MHC Class I	–		

*Demonstration of amyloid or other protein accumulation by established methods (e.g. for amyloid Congo red, crystal violet, thioflavin T/S, for other proteins p62, SMI-31, TDP-43). FF, finger flexion; HF, hip flexion; KE, knee extension; SA, shoulder abduction; MHC Class I, major histocompatibility complex class I; ULN, upper limit of normal.

Reproduced from Machado P et al. 'Sporadic inclusion body myositis: new insights and potential therapy.' *Curr Opin Neurol*; **27**(5): 2014: 591–8. PMC. Web. 8 May 2017 with permission from Wolters Kluwer Inc.

However, the aetiopathogenesis of IBM remains unresolved, and better animal models of IBM are clearly required.

Treatment

Evidence-based treatment recommendations cannot be made in IBM. However, limited studies confirm that IBM is resistant to immunosuppressive drugs,

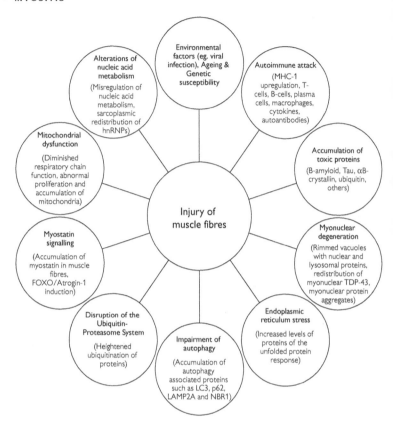

Figure 11.3 Potential pathogenic mechanisms leading to myofibre injury in inclusion body myositis.

Reproduced from Machado et al. 'Sporadic inclusion body myositis: new insights and potential therapy' *Curr Opin Neurol*; 2014; **27**(5): 591–8, with permission from Wolters Kluwer Health, Inc.

including: glucocorticoids, methotrexate, mycophenolate mofetil, ciclosporin, tacrolimus, intravenous immunoglobulins (IVIG), TNF-alpha blockers, and to ILI-blockers (anakinra). Trends towards improvement in dysphagia associated with IBM have been reported with IVIG, but such findings have never been replicated in adequately powered randomized-controlled trials (RCT).

With insufficient data for evidence-based treatment, some clinicians use steroids in cases with diagnostic doubt, and occasionally in younger patients with florid inflammation on biopsy. IVIG is sometimes used in rapidly deteriorating cases, or in patients with significant dysphagia. Patients with an associated connective tissue disease may show an initial response to immunosuppression.

Alemtuzumab infusions are capable of reducing T-cell infiltrates in IBM muscle biopsies, although no clear clinical improvements were demonstrated. Animal studies show that lithium can modulate tau phosphorylation via suppression of glycogen synthase kinase-3β, which could be of benefit in IBM; however, this potential benefit remains unproven in IBM. An open-label study with natalizumab (a humanized monoclonal antibody against the cell adhesion molecule α4-integrin) finished recruitment. (NCT02483845). A RDBPCT with rapamycin (an immunosuppressive and anticancer drug that acts by inhibiting target of rapamycin (TOR)) also recently finished enrolling IBM patients (NCT02481453).

Mounting evidence suggests that there is disruption of protein homeostasis in IBM, resulting from impaired protein degradation by the ubiquitin-proteasome system (UPS), which may underlie the characteristic degenerative pathology. Protein chaperones, such as heat shock protein 70 (HSP70), bind to aberrant proteins to prevent aggregation. An increase in HSP70 expression, and HSP70 and αB-crystallin immuno-reactivity in IBM inclusion bodies, suggests a diminished capacity of chaperone proteins in IBM. These findings suggest that approaches aimed at restoring protein homeostasis may be therapeutic in IBM. In a recent small RDBPCT, up-regulation of the heat shock response was tested by treatment with arimoclomol, an oral pharmacological agent that induces the synthesis of HSP70. In this trial, patients were randomized with a 2:1 arimoclomol:placebo ratio. The investigational drug was administered for 4 months, the arimoclomol dose being 100 mg TDS. After the 4-month treatment phase, an 8-month blinded follow-up phase followed. No major safety issues were observed and the drug was well tolerated. Efficacy measures were secondary outcomes. Numerically, the rate of decline in physical function (IBM functional rating scale) and muscle strength (right hand grip maximum voluntary isometric contraction testing and manual muscle testing) were less in the arimoclomol group compared to placebo, though the trend was not significant. A large RDBPCT with arimoclomol in IBM patients is expected soon (NCT02753530).

The myostatin pathway is a central negative regulator of myogenesis during development and periods of muscle regeneration in postnatal life, and its inhibition enhances muscle regeneration in animal models. Myostatin knockout mice have an increased muscle mass without organomegally and a range of animals, in addition to humans with loss of function mutations, show muscle hypertrophy with increased strength. This pathway thus represents a major target of interest for therapeutic manipulations in muscular conditions characterized by weakness and atrophy. A small RDBPCT with bimagrumab, an intravenously administered monoclonal antibody that binds competitively to activin receptor type IIB with greater affinity than myostatin, reported that the drug was well tolerated with significant improvements in muscle volume (measured by MRI) and lean body mass. A large bimagrumab study has completed, and recently published in abstract format - bimagrumab did not reach the primary endpoint of improving 6MWD or showed an improvement in muscle strength.

Another myostatin antagonist is currently being tested in IBM. This uses follistatin gene therapy (FS344) delivered by adeno-associated virus (AAV) and administered by quadriceps intramuscular injection. This trial is testing the safety of three different doses of AAV-FS344, and is measuring muscle strength, physical function, and thigh circumference. Muscle MRI and muscle histopathology are secondary study outcomes (NCT01519349).

Lack of restorative treatment for IBM means that exercise (e.g. aerobic exercise and strength training) has an important role in managing symptoms and minimizing physical capability loses. Although historically people with muscle conditions were advised not to exercise, for fear of inducing damage, recent studies have shown clear benefits of exercise without harm in neuromuscular conditions. Orthotic, and occupational and safety health interventions (e.g. house adaptations, falls prevention measures, etc.) should be made and tailored to each patient's needs. Advice from speech and language therapists should be available early for patients with dysphagia, who may need multidisciplinary support and more intensive therapeutic approaches when dysphagia becomes severe (e.g. oesophageal dilatation, cricopharyngeal myotomy, botulinum toxin injection into the upper oesophageal sphincter, and PEG feeding).

Conclusion

Despite recent advances, IBM aetiology remains unknown, and no pharmacological treatment has yet proven efficacious. However, research and pre-clinical experiments are ongoing, and the prospect of new clinical trials is encouraging. IBM is rare, so developing global strategies to foster research collaborations are crucial to improve diagnosis and treatment for this debilitating disease.

SUGGESTED READING

Ahmed M, Machado PM, Miller A, et al. (2016). Targeting protein homeostasis in sporadic inclusion body myositis. *Sci Transl Med*; **8**: 331ra41.

Askanas V, Engel WK, Nogalska A (2015). Sporadic inclusion-body myositis: a degenerative muscle disease associated with aging, impaired muscle protein homeostasis and abnormal mitophagy. *Biochim Biophys Acta*; **1852**: 633–43.

Benveniste O, Guiguet M, Freebody J, et al. (2011). Long-term observational study of sporadic inclusion body myositis. *Brain*; **134**: 3176–84.

Brady S, Healy EG, Machado P, Parton M, Holton JL, Hanna MG (2014). Inclusion body myositis: clinical review and current practice. *Clin Pract*; **11**: 623–37.

Cortese A, Machado P, Morrow J, et al. (2013). Longitudinal observational study of sporadic inclusion body myositis: implications for clinical trials. *Neuromuscul Disord*; **23**: 404–12.

Cox FM, Titulaer MJ, Sont JK, Wintzen AR, Verschuuren JJGM, Badrising UA (2011). A 12-year follow-up in sporadic inclusion body myositis: an end stage with major disabilities. *Brain*; **134**: 3167–75.

Dalakas MC (2015). Inflammatory muscle diseases. *N Engl J Med*; **372**: 1734–47.

Herbert MK, Pruijn GJ (2015). Novel serology testing for sporadic inclusion body myositis: disease-specificity and diagnostic utility. *Curr Opin Rheumatol*; **27**: 595–600.

Hilton-Jones D, Brady S (2016). Diagnostic criteria for inclusion body myositis. *J Intern Med*; **280**: 52–62.

Lloyd TE (2010). Novel therapeutic approaches for inclusion body myositis. *Curr Opin Rheumatol*; **22**: 658–64.

Machado PM, Ahmed, M, Brady S, et al. (2014). Ongoing developments in sporadic inclusion body myositis. *Curr Rheumatol Rep*; **16**: 477.

Machado PM, Dimachkie MM, Barohn RJ (2014). Sporadic inclusion body myositis: new insights and potential therapy. *Curr Opin Neurol*; **27**: 591–8.

Michelle EH, Mammen AL (2015). Myositis mimics. *Curr Rheumatol Rep*; **17**: 63.

Molberg O, Dobloug C (2016). Epidemiology of sporadic inclusion body myositis. *Curr Opin Rheumatol*, **28**: 657–60.

Morrow JM, Sinclair CD, Fischmann A, et al. (2016). MRI biomarker assessment of neuromuscular disease progression: a prospective observational cohort study. *Lancet Neurol*; **15**: 65–77.

Needham M, Mastaglia FL (2016). Sporadic inclusion body myositis: a review of recent clinical advances and current approaches to diagnosis and treatment. *Clin Neurophysiol*; **127**: 1764–73.

Phillips BA, Cala LA, Thickbroom GW, Melsom A, Zilko PJ, Mastaglia FL (2001). Patterns of muscle involvement in inclusion body myositis: clinical and magnetic resonance imaging study. *Muscle Nerve*; **24**: 1526–34.

Rose MR, Group EIW (2013). 188th ENMC International Workshop: Inclusion Body Myositis, 2–4 December 2011, Naarden, The Netherlands. *Neuromuscul Disord*; **23**: 1044–55.

Investigations

CHAPTER 12

Laboratory features—enzymes and biomarkers

Sarah L. Tansley and Neil J. McHugh

KEY POINTS

- CK is elevated in the majority of adult patients with myositis, but only 64% of children
- CK is useful for monitoring muscle disease activity
- Cardiac muscle damage in patients with idiopathic inflammatory myopathies (IIM) is best measured using troponin I
- Myositis specific or associated autoantibodies are identifiable in the majority patients, but rarely form part of routine laboratory 'autoimmune disease' screening panels. The most commonly identified autoantibodies varies between adult and juvenile onset disease
- Myositis specific and associated autoantibodies can divide patients into clinically useful and homogenous subgroups.

Skeletal muscle enzymes

What is creatine kinase?

Creatine kinase (CK) is a widely expressed enzyme responsible for the phosphorylation of creatine to phosphocreatine using adenosine triphosphate (ATP). In reverse, the reaction generates ATP, and phosphocreatine thereby acts as an energy repository and buffer for ATP during muscle rest.

CK is a dimer formed from B (brain) and M (muscle) subunits. There are three isoenzymes:

- CK MM (formed from two muscle subunits).
- CK BB (formed from two brain subunits).
- CK MB (formed from one muscle and one brain subunit).

CK isoenzyme expression patterns differ between tissues. In skeletal muscle 98% is the isotype CK-MM and approximately 1% CK-MB. In the myocardium approximately 70% is CK-MM and 25–30% CK-MB. In contrast in the brain and smooth muscle CK-BB is predominantly expressed.

Creatine kinase in patients with idiopathic inflammatory myopathies

Sarcoplasmic membrane muscle enzymes including CK are released following muscle cell damage in IIM and act as a marker for ongoing muscle destruction and regeneration. CK is considered the most sensitive of these enzymes; being elevated in the vast majority of adults with IIM and generally displaying the highest elevation above the normal range. CK level is typically higher in patients with polymyositis (PM) than dermatomyositis (DM), presumably reflecting the often greater degree of muscle involvement in patients with PM, but conversely is typically normal or only mildly elevated in those with inclusion body myositis (IBM).

CK is useful for disease monitoring in IIM and levels show a good overall correlation with disease activity and muscle strength. However, normal CK can occur in the context of active muscle disease; as indicated by persistent weakness and evidence of inflammation on muscle biopsy or magnetic resonance imaging. This may be due to either the suppression of CK release by prednisolone, the presence of circulating CK inhibitors and/or extensive muscle atrophy.

The isoenzyme CK-MM is the most sensitive and specific enzyme marker for skeletal muscle damage. However, CK-MB, which is usually a hallmark of acute myocardial injury, can also be elevated in IIM in the absence of cardiac disease. In this scenario elevated levels of CK-MB are thought to result from chronic skeletal muscle regeneration. It is important to remember therefore that detectable CK-MB and/or an elevated CK-MB/ total CK ratio do not always imply myocardial damage in the context of IIM.

Other causes of elevated CK are reviewed in Chapter 7.

Other skeletal muscle enzymes

In addition to CK other serum muscle enzymes including aspartate aminotransferase (AST), lactate dehydrogenase (LDH), alanine amino-transferase (ALT), and aldolase are often elevated in DM and PM, albeit less often and to a lesser extent than CK. ALT and AST are commonly referred to as 'liver function tests', although these enzymes are expressed in a variety of other tissues, including muscle. It is not unheard of for patients found to have an elevated ALT/AST to have a variety of other investigations, including liver biopsy before a diagnosis of myositis is considered. Once a diagnosis of myositis has been made this also has implications for disease monitoring, as in a patient with active disease elevated ALT/AST are more likely to be reflective of ongoing muscle inflammation than drug-induced toxicity; particularly when CK is also elevated.

Skeletal muscle enzymes in juvenile onset disease

In patients with juvenile-onset myositis, elevated skeletal muscle enzymes can be identified in approximately 80% (McCann et al. 2006). Unlike in adults, CK is not so ubiquitously increased and has been shown to be elevated in just 64% at diagnosis (McCann et al. 2006). Elevated LDH is more common and is identifiable in around three quarters of affected children. Elevation of ALT/AST is detectable in just under half of patients (McCann et al. 2006). CK may also be less helpful for disease monitoring in juvenile myositis, as levels have been shown to fall rapidly in response to treatment and remain low despite clinical evidence of ongoing disease activity (McCann et al. 2006). In another study increased levels of LDH and AST, but not CK or ALT, were found in relation to disease flares (Guzman et al. 1994). In juvenile-onset myositis it is therefore common practice to measure a range of skeletal muscle enzymes, rather than rely on CK alone.

Troponin

The troponins regulate the thin filament system in both cardiac and striated muscle. They each exist in three different isoforms, and both cardiac troponins I and T are considered highly specific markers of myocardial injury. Their measurement in suspected acute coronary syndrome has transformed the management of this disease and they are attractive biomarkers for detecting primary cardiac involvement in IIM, which is increasingly being recognized.

Caution is needed, however, as unlike cardiac troponin I, which is never expressed in skeletal muscle, troponin T is expressed in small amounts in developing foetal muscle development, healthy adults, and regenerating skeletal muscle of patients with IIM and muscular dystrophy (Aggarwal et al. 2009). Furthermore, cardiac troponin T has been found to be elevated in a significant proportion (41%) of patients with IIM with no apparent myocardial involvement (Erlacher et al. 2001). In patients with IIM, cardiac troponin T measurement has been found to correlate with skeletal muscle damage markers, including CK. This suggests that it may be a sensitive biomarker for low grade skeletal muscle inflammation in patients with IIM, but in this setting also does not necessarily reflect myocardial ischaemia or inflammation. (Erlacher et al. 2001). Cardiac muscle damage in patients with IIM is best measured using troponin I (Aggarwal et al. 2009).

General points

Laboratories often differ in their assay used, normal range, and test reproducibility. Where a test is to be used for disease monitoring it is important that the result is interpreted in the context of the patient, the laboratory, and the previous result.

While elevations of CK-MB and/or cardiac troponin T in patients with IIM do not necessarily imply cardiac involvement or myocardial damage, it is our opinion that cardiac disease should be actively excluded in these individuals.

Muscle specific and associated autoantibodies

Myositis specific and associated autoantibodies, and serological subsets of myositis

Myositis specific autoantibodies (MSA) are a collection of autoantibodies directed against intracellular antigens exclusively found in patients with IIM.

Myositis associated autoantibodies (MAA) can be identified in patients with myositis and also in those with other associated connective tissue disorders. Collectively these autoantibodies can be identified in approximately 80% adults and 60% children with myositis. They can identify homogenous subsets, and have both diagnostic and prognostic value. MSA/MAA can also be helpful in identifying those patients presenting with associated connective tissue diseases, such as scleroderma, that are at risk of developing muscle involvement and in identifying those patients with IIM who initially present without muscle disease. A particularly important group are those presenting with apparently 'idiopathic' interstitial lung disease (ILD) where the identification of a MSA will affect both treatment options and prognosis. Anti-synthetase autoantibodies for example have been identified in 7% of adult patients diagnosed with idiopathic ILD (Tansley and McHugh 2014).

For a summary of autoantibody associated clinical features see Table 12.1.

The same autoantibodies are seen in both adult and juvenile forms of myositis, and associations between Human Leucocyte Antigen (HLA) risk alleles and auto-antibody subgroups are common across the age range, suggesting similarities in the underlying pathogenesis. The frequency of MSA sub-groups, however, varies between adult and juvenile disease, and the population studied. The specific disease phenotype for autoantibody subgroups also varies depending on the population studied and between adults, children, and even young adults. It remains unclear whether the autoantibodies themselves contribute to pathology and, if so, how age and ethnic background/ environmental specific effects are mediated.

Myositis specific and associated autoantibody detection

Standard screening for autoantibodies in patients with rheumatological conditions typically starts with indirect immunofluorescence of HEp-2 cells looking for a positive anti-nuclear antibody (ANA) followed by further screening for extractable nuclear antigens (ENA) if positive, and using a standard panel of antigens. This approach is of limited value in patients with myositis as whilst up to 80% of patients will have a positive ANA this is frequently non-specific, and most MSA and MAA are not included as part of a standard ENA panel. Furthermore, a negative ANA result does not preclude the presence of a MSA, many of which produce cytoplasmic staining patterns.

The pattern seen on immunofluorescence can occasionally be helpful as cytoplasmic staining in a patient with myositis suggests the presence of an anti-synthetase autoantibody or anti-SRP, and a homogenous-nucleolar staining pattern should raise suspicion of anti-PmScl.

While MSA are typically mutually exclusive, the identification of a MAA such as anti-Ro does not preclude the presence of a more specific MSA and further testing is still warranted. Anti-Ro52 has been identified in conjunction with anti-Jo-1 in >50% of cases (Tansley and McHugh 2014).

Immunoprecipitation is generally considered the gold standard method for MSA detection, but is only available in a limited number of centres worldwide. A variety

Table 12.1 Myositis specific and associated autoantibody syndromes		
	Frequency	Associated clinical phenotype
Myositis specific autoantibodies		
Anti-synthetases[a]	Most common MSA in adult cohorts: anti-Jo-1 in 20–30% and others in 10–20%. Much rarer in juvenile onset (<5%) and typically found in older children.	Anti-synthetase syndrome: myositis, ILD, Raynaud's, mechanic's hands, Gottron's, arthritis, and pyrexia. Patient's may present with ILD and may never develop myositis—More likely if non-Jo-1 autoantibodies. ILD is a major cause of mortality.
Anti-Mi2	Approximately 10%	Classic DM that typically responds well to standard treatment.
Anti-TIF1γ	15–20% adult and 20–30% juvenile onset	Severe skin disease often in a photosensitive distribution. Red on white lesions. Associated with lipodystrophy in juvenile onset and malignancy in adults.
Anti-NXP2	Varies widely with cohort studied. Common in juvenile onset 20–25%	Calcinosis, a greater degree of weakness and severe disease in juvenile onset and possible malignancy in adults.
Anti-MDA5	Common (>30%) of East Asian cohorts and ~10% Caucasian myositis populations.	Clinically amyopathic DM or less severe muscle involvement. ILD and rapidly progressive ILD with high associated mortality in East Asian cohorts. Characteristic cutaneous phenotype with ulceration.
Anti-SAE	Rare	Initially amyopathic DM but progresses to muscle involvement.
Anti-SRP	Rare. ~5% adults and less in juvenile-onset.	Necrotizing immune myositis with markedly elevated CK and severe weakness. Additional features include dysphagia, cardiac involvement and arthritis. May be treatment refractory.
Anti-HMGCR	Rare. ~6% adults	Necrotizing immune myositis associated with statin use. 40–60% have no history of statin exposure. May be treatment refractory.

continued >

Table 12.1 Myositis specific and associated autoantibody syndromes

(continued)

	Frequency	Associated clinical phenotype
Myositis-associated autoantibodies		
Anti-Ro52	Found alongside anti-Jo-1 in >50% of cases. ~6% juvenile onset.	Uncertain. Possible more severe ILD.
Anti-PmScl	~4% juvenile-onset	Polymyositis–scleroderma overlap. Limited cutaneous scleroderma, muscle disease, ILD, and calcinosis. Similarities with anti-synthetase syndrome.
Anti-U1-RNP	~6% juvenile-onset	Myositis overlap CTD.
Anti-Ku		Myositis overlap CTD.
Anti-cytoplasmic 5′-nucleotidase 1	Identifiable in 30–75% of sporadic IBM	Also identified in Sjögrens syndrome, SLE, and rarely in other myositis subtypes.

ᵃ Jo-1, PL12, PL7, OJ, EJ, KS, Zo, Ha.

Data sourced from Tansley SL, McHugh NJ. Myositis specific and associated autoantibodies in the diagnosis and management of juvenile and adult idiopathic inflammatory myopathies. *Curr Rheumatol Rep*; 2014;**16**(12): 464; and Lloyd TE, Christopher-Stine L, Pinal-Fernandez I et al. 'Cytosolic 5′-nucleotidase 1A is a common target of circulating autoantibodies in several autoimmune diseases'. *Arthritis Care Res*; 2016; **68**: 66–71.

of different immunological assays have been designed to detect MSA in the research setting and multiplex assays using the same technologies have also been developed with the advantage of being able to detect many specific autoantibodies simultaneously. Several multiplex kits are now commercially available that contain a panel of MSA, including those relevant to juvenile-onset disease. Such methods will only detect the specific panel autoantibodies screened for, and clinicians must be aware of what is and is not included. As with all new technology it remains important to ensure that new assays are appropriately validated; ensuring the ANA pattern on immunofluorescence is consistent with the autoantibody result obtained can be helpful in identifying potential false positive or otherwise erroneous results.

The development of quantitative and semi-quantitative techniques to detect myositis specific autoantibodies has led to a growing interest in the potential clinical utility of autoantibody titre to predict disease activity and response to treatment. In adults, small studies have shown a relationship between the titres of anti-Jo-1, anti-MDA5, anti-HMGCR, and anti-SRP autoantibodies with disease activity measures (Stone et al. 2007; Benveniste et al. 2011; Muro et al. 2012; Werner et al. 2012). In addition, the titre of anti-MDA5 has been shown to be useful in predicting response to treatment in Japanese children with JDM.

Other biomarkers

A significant limitation of the tests described above is their inability to reliably indicate disease activity or response to treatment. Muscle enzymes can be insensitive in this regard and, like muscle strength, are affected by muscle damage and do not assess extra-muscular disease manifestations. Autoantibody titre has shown promise as a means of disease monitoring, but at this stage data is very limited.

Cytokines, the interferon signature and disease activity

A variety of cytokines have been systematically investigated as potential biomarkers for disease monitoring in IIM and many including IL-6, IL-8, CXCL-10, CXC3CLI, TNF-α, BAFF, and IP-10 show correlations with measures of disease activity. The Interferon signature refers to an 'immune fingerprint' of genes and chemokines up regulated by interferon, including IL-6, IL-8, and TNFα. Scores based on serum levels of various components of the interferon signature and have shown correlation with changes in global myositis disease activity in both affected adults and children (Reed et al. 2012). Interferon peripheral blood gene 'scores' may thus act as useful longitudinal markers of change in disease activity. Furthermore, scores in combination with autoantibody subgroup may help predict the response to medications like Rituximab (Reed et al. 2015).

Biomarkers and interstitial lung disease

Some cytokines may be useful in identifying associated ILD in patients with IIM, and assessing the progression and severity of pulmonary fibrosis once the diagnosis has been established. Many of the potential biomarkers investigated in this regard are not unique to myositis associated ILD and may be increased in a wide range of pulmonary diseases including various types of ILD. Raised levels of IL-6, IL-8, TNF-α, and IP-10 have been found in subsets of myositis patients with ILD, and levels reduce following appropriate treatment. IL-6 levels have been shown to predict the prognosis of clinically amyopathic dermatomyositis patients with rapidly progressive ILD.

Other promising biomarkers for ILD in myositis include the glycoprotein KL-6 (krebs von lungen-6) and SP-D (surfactant protein D), both secreted by type II alveolar epithelial cells. Increased levels reflect alveolar injury, and can be useful in assessing disease activity, treatment response and prognosis. Serum ferritin has also been suggested as a marker of ILD severity, particularly in patients with rapidly-progressive ILD, and levels have been shown to correlate with disease activity and prognosis.

Urinary myoglobin

Myoglobin released from inflamed or damaged muscle can be detected in the urine. In myositis the degree of myoglobinuria is usually insufficient to lead to urine discolouration, so called 'coca cola urine', but can be detected by dip stick analysis. This does not typically form part of routine clinical assessment of a patient with suspected myositis, but is noteworthy in view of the fact that the presence of urinary myoglobin may lead to a false positive result for haematuria on urinalysis: Thus, haematuria in the absence of urinary red cells can provide an important clue for the presence of muscle disease in a patient with non-specific symptoms.

REFERENCES

Aggarwal R, Lebiedz-Odrobina D, Sinha A, Manadan A, Case JP. (2009). Serum cardiac troponin T, but not troponin I, is elevated in idiopathic inflammatory myopathies. *J Rheumatol*; **36**: 2711–14.

Benveniste O, Drouot L, Jouen F, et al. (2011). Correlation of anti-signal recognition particle autoantibody levels with creatine kinase activity in patients with necrotizing myopathy. *Arthritis Rheum*; **63**: 1961–71.

Erlacher P, Lercher A, Falkensammer J, et al. (2001). Cardiac troponin and beta-type myosin heavy chain concentrations in patients with polymyositis or dermatomyositis. *Clin Chim Acta*; **306**: 27–33.

Guzman J, Petty RE, Malleson PN. (1994). Monitoring disease activity in juvenile dermatomyositis: the role of von Willebrand factor and muscle enzymes. *J Rheumatol*; **21**: 739–43.

Lloyd TE, Christopher-Stine L, Pinal-Fernandez I, et al. (2016). Cytosolic 5'-nucleotidase 1A is a common target of circulating autoantibodies in several autoimmune diseases. *Arthritis Care Res (Hoboken)*; **68**: 66–71.

McCann LJ, Juggins AD, Maillard SM, et al. (2006). The Juvenile Dermatomyositis National Registry and Repository (UK and Ireland)—clinical characteristics of children recruited within the first 5 yr. *Rheumatol (Oxf)*; **45**: 1255–60.

Muro Y, Sugiura K, Hoshino K, Akiyama M. (2012). Disappearance of anti-MDA-5 autoantibodies in clinically amyopathic DM/interstitial lung disease during disease remission. *Rheumatol (Oxf)*; **51**: 800–4.

Reed AM, Crowson CS, Hein M, et al. (2015). Biologic predictors of clinical improvement in rituximab-treated refractory myositis. *BMC Musculoskel Disord*; **16**: 257.

Reed AM, Peterson E, Bilgic H, et al. (2012). Changes in novel biomarkers of disease activity in juvenile and adult dermatomyositis are sensitive biomarkers of disease course. *Arthritis Rheum*; **64**: 4078–86.

Stone KB, Oddis CV, Fertig N, Katsumata Y, Lucas M, Vogt M, et al. (2007). Anti-Jo-1 antibody levels correlate with disease activity in idiopathic inflammatory myopathy. *Arthritis Rheum*; **56**: 3125–31.

Tansley SL, McHugh NJ. (2014). Myositis specific and associated autoantibodies in the diagnosis and management of juvenile and adult idiopathic inflammatory myopathies. *Curr Rheumatol Rep*; **16**: 464.

Werner JL, Christopher-Stine L, Ghazarian SR, et al. (2012). Antibody levels correlate with creatine kinase levels and strength in anti-3-hydroxy-3-methylglutaryl-coenzyme A reductase-associated autoimmune myopathy. *Arthritis Rheum*; **64**: 4087–93.

CHAPTER 13

Histopathological features of the idiopathic inflammatory myopathies

Marianne de Visser and Eleonora M.A. Aronica

KEY POINTS

- In adult patients with presummed IIM, a muscle biopsy is mandatory to confirm the diagnosis and exclude a myopathy which would not respond to glucocorticoids or other immunosuppressants, including inclusion body myositis (IBM)

- The optimal biopsy technique is that which is regularly used by an individual expert in IIM patient care, and includes open and percutaneous techniques, the latter under local anaesthetic

- Imaging guides muscle biopsy site, targeting affected muscles, and avoiding those with end- stage damage

- The laboratory skill level required to adequately interrogate muscle samples histologically and immuno-histochemically dictates that this work should be undertaken only in dedicated facilities with appropriate expertise

- A standardized set of laboratory stains has been agreed internationally to interrogate muscle samples obtained from presumed IIM patients

- Histological features may differentiate between IIM subgroups

- In patients with a polymyositis (PM) phenotype, but who remain treatment-resistant, early clinical reassessment, and repeat biopsy should be considered

- Repeat biopsies are not usual for monitoring purposes, except in the research setting

- In patients with clinically overt IBM of recent onset, diagnostic pathological changes may be absent

- Necrotizing immune-mediated myopathy is usually not associated with significant inflammation.

Introduction

The adult IIM include dermatomyositis (DM), polymyositis (PM), immune-mediated necrotizing myopathy (IMNM), overlap myositis associated with connective tissue disease (CTD), antisynthetase syndrome (ASS) associated with myositis, and inclusion body myositis (IBM). Most IIM are usually if variably treatment responsive, whereas immunosuppression and immunomodulatory regimes do not alter IBM outcomes. First line therapy for IIM, other than IBM, usually includes long-term corticosteroids and at relatively high-doses, a regime fraught with iatrogenic dangers. To avoid inappropriate corticosteroid use in IBM, and other non-immune mediated myopathies, making an accurate diagnosis is clearly of paramount importance. IIM diagnosis is based on clinical, laboratory, and histopathological examinations. The diagnostic utility of muscle enzymes, myositis serology, electromyography, and magnetic resonance imaging are discussed elsewhere in this handbook.

Except for patients with the highly characteristic skin changes of DM, or where myositis occurs in association with a proven other CTD, a muscle biopsy is considered mandatory to confirm an IIM diagnosis, and to definitively exclude other myopathies capable of mimicking an IIM. IIM clearly represent a heterogeneous disease spectrum, with subtypes distinguishable by characteristic clinical features and muscle specific serology. Whether serologically defined IIM subtypes have specific histopathological associations remains to be determined. There is debate regarding the need for a muscle biopsy for diagnosing IBM. Previously a definite IBM diagnosis was defined on histopathological features, consisting of an inflammatory myopathy with mononuclear cell invasion of non-necrotic muscle fibres, vacuolated fibres, and either intracellular amyloid deposits or 15–18 nm tubulofilaments visualized by electron microscopy (Griggs et al. 1995). However, the sensitivity of these histological criteria for a definite IBM diagnosis was found to be very low. Only one of these pathological features is needed to meet 'clinically-defined' criteria in patients with a typical pattern of muscle weakness (knee extensor ≥ hip flexor and finger flexor ≥ shoulder abduction (Rose 2013). Subsequently, these clinical criteria were also found to have relatively low sensitivity, in particular many patients failed to meet 'knee extensor weakness > hip flexor weakness'. A relatively simple further set of criteria has been proposed, with 90% sensitivity and 96% specificity, using the following three criteria combined: finger flexor OR quadriceps weakness, endomysial inflammation with invasion of non-necrotic muscle fibres OR rimmed vacuoles (Lloyd et al. 2014). Despite that the diagnosis of IBM is made clinically, by history, and thorough neurological examination, muscle biopsy findings are considered as supportive or confirmatory, so clinicians still rely on muscle histology.

Selection of muscle biopsy

Muscle biopsies should be taken from a muscle which is symptomatic, usually the quadriceps or the deltoid. Muscle biopsy results are diagnostically inconclusive in 10–20% of cases, due to sampling error caused by the patchy distribution of inflammatory infiltrates, even when the muscle biopsied was clinically weak. It is important to avoid undertaking a biopsy of a muscle that has undergone recent needle electromyography. Muscle imaging may optimize biopsy site selection, as muscle magnetic resonance imaging can demonstrate muscle oedema on fat-suppressed short tau inversion recovery (STIR), even in clinically asymptomatic muscles (Van de Vlekkert et al. 2015). It is best to avoid biopsying a severely affected muscle, as end stage changes may render the biopsy non-diagnostic.

Biopsy technique and tissue preparation

In order to increase the diagnostic yield, muscle specimens can be obtained by an open surgical technique, which allows for acquisition of potentially larger samples, though clinicians may prefer to use percutaneous techniques, such as the conchotome forceps or the Bergström needle, conducted under local anaesthesia. In children, and rarely in some adults, general anaesthesia may be required. There is a very small risk of haemorrhage and/or infection. Following open procedures, it is not uncommon to have a patch of numbness around the scar. Obtained muscle specimens are usually approximately 1 × 0.5 × 0.5 cm in size. Following their excision, samples are transported (placed on gauze lightly dampened with saline) to the laboratory for processing. Additional samples can be obtained through the same incision and fixed in glutaraldehyde, to enable future electron microscopy.

Histochemical and (immuno)histochemical studies are performed on frozen material. To prevent ice crystal artefact and ensure an optimal preservation of enzyme activity, the specimen is snap frozen in isopentane cooled in liquid nitrogen to –160°C, either before or after mounting the sample on a piece of cork by a small amount of embedding compound for cryosectioning (Tissue-Tek OCT). Sections 6–10 μm are cut and stained with a panel of (immuno)histochemical stains. If the specimen is > 0.8 cm long, part of the material can be fixed in formalin for routine histopathology. The glutaraldehyde-fixed specimen for electron microscopy is post-fixed with 1% osmiumtetroxide, block-stained with 1% uranyl acetate, dehydrated in dimethoxypropane and embedded in epoxyresin. Semi-thin sections (1–2 μm) are stained with toluidine blue and examined under oil immersion optics.

Panel of (immuno)histochemical stains recommended for diagnosis of idiopathic inflammatory myopathies

Table 13.1 shows the panel of stains that are routinely used for the pathological examination of all IIM subtypes. This selection is the result of a consensus meeting in which a large international group with significant expertise in reading of muscle biopsies from suspected IIM patients participated (De Bleecker et al. 2015). Many were concerned that performing a limited set of stains with a high yield in IIM may not sufficiently exclude other neuromuscular diseases, and suggested that a basic panel of stains should be done in each biopsy.

Table 13.1 Recommended list of diagnostic stains on muscle biopsy specimens in IIMs

Required stains	Additional stains for suspected IIM	Optional stains for suspected IIM
H&E	AK	CD20/CD79a
ATPases/myosin F/S	CD3, CD8, CD68	CD4
NADH	HLA-ABC/MHC-I	CD138
SDH	MAC (c5b-9)	BDCA1/BDCA2
COX or COX/SDH	p62	HLA-DR/MHC-II
Gomori's trichrome	CD31	TDP43
PAS		CD56/NCAM
Oro/Sudan black		Myosin-foetal
AP		
NE		
Congo red		

Reproduced from De Bleecker et al., 205th ENMC International Workshop: Pathology diagnosis of idiopathic inflammatory myopathies Part II (2014). *Neuromuscul Disord*; **25**: 268–272 with permission from Elsevier.

Abbreviations: AK, alkaline phosphatase; AP, acid phosphatase; (F/S) fast/slow; COX, cytochrome c oxidase; H&E, haematoxylin and eosin; IIM, idiopathic inflammatory myopathy; MAC, membrane attack complex; NADH, nicotinamide adenine dinucleotide dehydrogenase-tetrazolium reductase; NCAM, neural cell adhesion molecule; NE, non-specific esterase; ORO, Oil-red-O; SDH, succinate dehydrogenase.

BDCA1 and BDCA2 stain myeloid and plasmacytoid dendritic cells, respectively.

MHC, major histocompatibility complex; PAS, periodic acid-Schiff; TDP43, TAR DNA-binding protein 43.

Histopathological features of various subtypes of idiopathic inflammatory myopathies

Dermatomyositis

The International Juvenile Dermatomyositis Biopsy Consensus Group designed and tested a scoring tool for the assessment of the nature and severity of pathological changes in biopsy specimens from patients with suspected or proven juvenile dermatomyositis (JDM) (Wedderburn et al. 2007). This tool assesses features characteristic of JDM, organized into four domains (inflammatory, vascular, muscle fibre, and connective tissue). The tool was proven to have high inter- and intra-observer agreements, and can be used on biceps and quadriceps muscle tissues. The tool also proved to correlate well with clinical measures of disease activity (Varsani et al. 2015). In juvenile and adult DM, muscle biopsies typically demonstrate inflammatory infiltrates of mainly CD4+ T cells, but with macrophages, plasmacytoid dendritic cells and CD20+ B cells, which are confined to the perimysium, often around blood vessels, with perifascicular muscle fibre atrophy (Figure 13.1A), and scattered necrotic and regenerating fibres (Arahata and Engel 1984). Major histocompatibility complex type I (MHC I) is upregulated in perifascicular muscle fibres (Figure 13.1B). The earliest demonstrable abnormality in DM is deposition of the C5b-9 complement membrane attack complex (MAC) on small blood vessels (Emslie-Smith and Engel 1990). MAC deposition precedes inflammation and other structural abnormalities particularly in the perifascicular region.

The subsequent necrosis of small blood vessels causes a reduction in capillary density. Perifascicular atrophy is invariably associated with capillary depletion. MAC deposits in capillaries result from activation of the classical complement pathway, triggered by the direct binding of C1q to damaged capillaries. Perifascicular atrophy is not found in amyopathic DM, but is present in 40–90% of adult DM patients. In children, perifascicular atrophy is observed in ~75% of JDM cases.

Sarcoplasmic myxovirus resistance (MxA) expression detected by immunohistochemistry is a more sensitive marker of DM than perifascicular atrophy and MAC deposition on endomysial capillaries (Uruha et al. 2017).

At the ultrastructural level, DM angiopathy is characterized by endothelial necrosis, leading to destruction of the vascular wall and platelet thrombi, with subsequent endothelial regeneration. A characteristic finding early in the disease process is the presence of tubuloreticular inclusions in endothelial cells, often preceding inflammatory cell infiltrates. These inclusions are related to the endoplasmatic reticulum or to the outer nuclear membrane of the endothelial cell and are considered downstream markers of type I interferon signalling (De Visser et al. 1989; Greenberg 2011).

As in muscle, the typical cutaneous histopathologic changes in dermal DM are indicative of microvascular injury, including vascular C5–9 deposition, minimal inflammation, endothelial injury, occlusive fibrin thrombi, and hypovascularity. Fasciitis manifesting with inflammatory infiltrates with CD4+ T-cells and CD20+ B-cells around the fascial small blood vessels is found in nearly all DM patients, even when amyopathic. Panniculitis can occur, although only rarely.

Overlap myositis

Overlap myositis is defined as an IIM occurring in association with an established other CTD. If autoantibodies are present these are usually myositis-associated antibodies, e.g. anti-SSA (Ro), anti-RNP, anti-Scl70, etc. (Troyanov et al. 2014). In overlap myositis the histopathological picture often resembles that of DM, with perivascular cell infiltrates, albeit predominantly composed of macrophages (Figure 13.1C–E). As for DM, muscle fibre pathology may occur in perifascicular regions. Tubuloreticular inclusions in endothelial cells can be found in a proportion of overlap cases.

Antisynthetase syndrome

Pathology in the perimysium and neighbouring muscle fibres is the hallmark histo-pathology in ASS. A prominent feature is the presence of necrotic and regen-erating fibres, which strongly cluster in perifascicular regions (Figure 13.1F). Sarcolemmal complement deposition is restricted to perifascicular fibres. MHC I staining is diffusely positive, but particularly in perifascicular areas. Cellular infiltrates are mainly located in the perimysium and/or around vessels, often extending into the endomysium. Endomysial lymphocytes invading or surround-ing non-necrotic fibres are usually present. Inflammation is associated with peri-mysial fragmentation, highlighted by alkaline phosphatase staining (Figure 13.1F and G). CD68+ macrophages are abundant and, in addition, T cells (CD4+ cells and CD8+ cells), and to a lesser extent CD20+ B cells are also observed. The macrophages and CD8+ cells can also be found in the endomysium. ASS and DM share some histopathological features. Myofibre necrosis in perifascicular regions and perimysial fragmentation can also be found in DM, but not as prominently as in ASS, whereas signs of vasculopathy, i.e. C5b-9 capillary deposits, microtubular inclusions, and capillary depletion may be present in ASS, but to a lesser extent as compared to DM.

Immune-mediated necrotizing myopathy

Muscle histology from anti-SRP (signal recognition particle) or HMGCR (3-hydroxy-3-methylglutaryl-coenzyme A reductase) antibody positive or sero-negative IMNM cases is characterized by the presence of necrotic muscle fibres as the predominant histological abnormality, distributed randomly across the biopsy specimen (Figure 13.1H). There is sparse macrophage- predominant, lymphocyte-poor infiltration of inflammatory cells with sometimes prominent endomysial fibrosis. Deposition of MAC on small blood vessels or thickened basement membrane (pipestem capillaries) may be seen at the ultrastructural level, but tubuloreticular inclusions in endothelial cells are uncommon or not evident. Sarcolemmal MHC I expression is variable.

Polymyositis—separate entity or inclusion body myositis phenotype?

As for IBM, mononuclear cells in PM are usually located in the endomysium and consist of predominantly CD8+ T lymphocytes, plasma cells, myeloid dendritic cells, and macrophages. The lymphocytes surround and also invade non-necrotic muscle fibres that express MHC I on the sarcolemma. Thus, PM appears to be the result of an MHC I-restricted cytotoxic T-cell response against an (auto)antigen expressed by muscle fibres (Dalakas 2015). The finding of MHC overexpression and CD8+ T cells (termed the MHC–CD8 complex) is not only useful for confirming the diagnosis, but also for ruling out disorders without primary inflammation, such as some muscular dystrophies (Hoogendijk et al. 2004). Currently, there is much debate regarding the existence of PM as

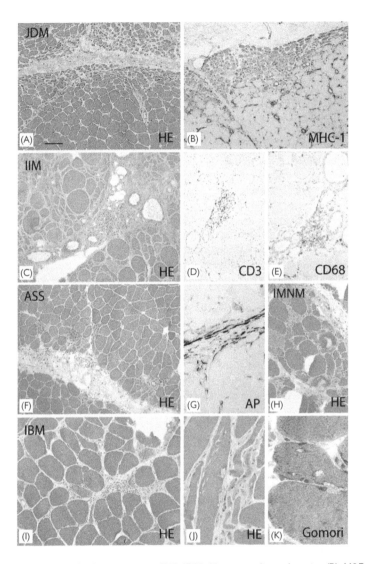

Figure 13.1 *Juvenile dermatomyositis* [(A) JDM, Haematoxylin and eosin; (B) H&E, major histocompatibility complex class I, MHC-1] showing perifascicular atrophy. *Non-specific* or *overlap myositis* (NSM/OM) in a patient with rheumatoid myositis [(C) H&E; (D) CD3; (E) CD68)] showing a perimysial perivascular cell infiltrate composed of CD3-positive lymphocytes and macrophages. *Antisynthetase syndrome* [ASS; (F) H&E; (G) alkaline phosphatase, AP] showing the presence of necrotic and regenerating fibres strongly clustered in perifascicular regions, and fragmentation of the perimysium staining intensely with AP. *Immune-mediated necrotizing myopathy (IMNM)*; (H) H&E, showing necrotic muscle fibres and no significant inflammation. Inclusion body myositis (I) H&E showing an endomysial cell infiltrate invading a non-necrotic muscle fibre and rimmed vacuoles (J) H&E; (K) modified trichrome Gomori. Scale bar in A: (A–F) 80 mM; (G–J) 40 mM; (K) 20 mM. See Colour Plate Section.

a separate entity (Van der Meulen et al. 2003; Troyanov et al. 2014; Vilela et al. 2015). Histopathologically defined PM shows a picture consistent with IBM, save for the absence of rimmed vacuoles. If such a histopathological picture is found, one should be cautious and actively search for clinical features confirmatory of IBM, including asymmetry, weakness of distal muscles (finger flexors and tibialis anterior muscle).

Inclusion body myositis

IBM muscle pathology typically demonstrates extensive endomysial inflammation, with inflammatory cells composed of macrophages and CD8+ cytotoxic/suppressor lymphocytes surrounding non-necrotizing myofibres expressing MHC-I on the sarcolemma as in PM (Figure 13.1I). Of note, MHC-I expression is also seen in non-inflammatory disorders, and combined use of MHC-I and MHC-II staining has been suggested to increase the specificity for IIMs, and particularly for IBM. In addition, in IBM there are often end-stage myopathic features with increases in connective tissue, variability in fibre size, autophagic vacuoles that have walls lined internally with material that stains bluish-red with haematoxylin and eosin or modified Gomori trichrome (Figures 13.1J and 13.1K), 'ragged-red' or cytochrome oxidase–negative fibres representing abnormal mitochondria and congophilic amyloid deposits next to the vacuoles. Electron microscopy shows tubulofilaments 15–18 nm in diameter next to the vacuoles (Griggs et al. 1995).

There is an ongoing debate regarding whether the presence of rimmed vacuoles is required for the diagnosis of IBM. IBM patients with characteristic clinical features may have muscle histology showing endomysial CD8+ lymphocytes invading non-necrotic muscle fibres, but without rimmed vacuoles, even in repeat biopsies. A recent study has convincingly shown that there is no difference in disease course or treatment response in IBM patients fulfilling histopathological criteria and those who fulfil clinical, but not all histopathological, criteria (Brady et al. 2013). Given the low sensitivity of rimmed vacuoles, other biomarkers have been sought. LC3 and p62 were found to be sensitive autophagic markers of IBM. Aggregation-prone protein TAR-DNA binding protein-43 (TDP-43) is highly specific, but has relatively low sensitivity for IBM (Hiniker et al. 2013).

Future directions

There is a need for additional histopathological studies on cohorts of patients based on clinical phenotype (site and severity of affected skeletal muscles, site and severity of skin changes, associated organ involvement, and cancer) and serological profile. As for JDM, consensus should be reached on the assessment of features histological characteristic of IIM subtypes, also organized into four domains (inflammatory, vascular, muscle fibre, and connective tissue). The design, evaluation, and subsequent fine-tuning of this assessment tool is currently in progress.

REFERENCES

Arahata K, Engel AG (1984). Monoclonal antibody analysis of mononuclear cells in myopathies. I: quantitation of subsets according to diagnosis and sites of accumulation and demonstration and counts of muscle fibers invaded by T cells. *Ann Neurol*; **16**: 193–208.

Brady S, Squier W, Hilton-Jones D (2013). Clinical assessment determines the diagnosis of inclusion body myositis independently of pathological features. *J Neurol Neurosurg Psychiatr*; **84**: 1240–6.

Dalakas MC (2015). Inflammatory muscle diseases. *N Engl J Med*; **372**: 1734–47.

De Bleecker JL, De Paepe B, Aronica E, et al. (2015). 205th ENMC International Workshop: Pathology diagnosis of idiopathic inflammatory myopathies part II 28–30 March 2014, Naarden, The Netherlands. *Neuromuscul Disord*; **25**: 268–72.

De Visser M, Emslie-Smith AM, Engel AG. (1989). Early ultrastructural alterations in adult dermatomyositis. Capillary abnormalities precede other structural changes in muscle. *J Neurol Sci*; **94**: 181–92.

Emslie-Smith AM, Engel AG (1990). Microvascular changes in early and advanced dermatomyositis: a quantitative study. *Ann Neurol*; **27**: 343–56.

Greenberg SA (2011). Inclusion body myositis. *Curr Opin Rheumatol*; **23**: 574–8.

Griggs RC, Askanas V, DiMauro S, et al. (1995). Inclusion body myositis and myopathies. *Ann Neurol*; **38**: 705–13.

Hiniker A, Daniels BH, Lee HS, Margeta M (2013). Comparative utility of LC3, p62 and TDP-43 immunohistochemistry in differentiation of inclusion body myositis from polymyositis and related inflammatory myopathies. *Acta Neuropath Commun*; **1**: 29.

Hoogendijk JE, Amato AA, Lecky BR, et al. (2004). 119th ENMC international workshop: trial design in adult idiopathic inflammatory myopathies, with the exception of inclusion body myositis, 10–12 October 2003, Naarden, the Netherlands. *Neuromuscul Disord*; **14**: 337–45.

Lloyd TE, Mammen AL, Amato AA, et al. (2014). Evaluation and construction of diagnostic criteria for inclusion body myositis. *Neurology*; **83**: 426–33.

Rose MR (2013). ENMC IBM Working Group. 188th ENMC International Workshop: Inclusion Body Myositis, 2–4 December 2011, Naarden, The Netherlands. *Neuromuscul Disord*; **23**: 1044–55.

Troyanov Y, Targoff IN, Payette MP, et al. (2014). Redefining dermatomyositis: a description of new diagnostic criteria that differentiate pure dermatomyositis from overlap myositis with dermatomyositis features. *Medicine (Balt)*; **93**: 318–32.

Uruha A, Nishikawa A, Tsuburaya RS, et al. (2017). Sarcoplasmic MxA expression: A valuable marker of dermatomyositis. *Neurology*; **88**: 493–500.

Van de Vlekkert J, Maas M, Hoogendijk JE, De Visser M, Van Schaik IN (2015). Combining MRI and muscle biopsy improves diagnostic accuracy in subacute-onset idiopathic inflammatory myopathy. *Muscle Nerve*; **51**: 253–8.

Van der Meulen MF, Bronner IM, Hoogendijk JE, et al. (2003). Polymyositis: an overdiagnosed entity. *Neurology*; **61**: 316–21.

Varsani H, Charman SC, Li CK, et al. (2015). Validation of a score tool for measurement of histological severity in juvenile dermatomyositis and association with clinical severity of disease. *Ann Rheum Dis*; **74**: 204–10.

Vilela VS, Prieto-González S, Milisenda JC, Selva-O Callaghan A, Grau JM (2015). Polymyositis, a very uncommon isolated disease: clinical and histological re-evaluation after long-term follow-up. *Rheumatol Int*; **35**: 915–20.

Wedderburn LR, Varsani H, Li CK, et al. (2007). International consensus on a proposed score system for muscle biopsy evaluation in patients with juvenile dermatomyositis: a tool for potential use in clinical trials. *Arthritis Rheum*; **57**: 1192–201.

CHAPTER 13

CHAPTER 14

Imaging of skeletal muscle

Nicolo Pipitone

KEY POINTS

- Multiple forms of imaging may be used to investigate a patient suspected of idiopathic inflammatory myopathy (IIM), each with different efficacies and specificities towards myositis symptoms
- Some forms of imaging, such as plain radiography and computed tomography (CT), are unsuitable for diagnostic and investigatory purposes when related to IIM
- Muscle magnetic resonance imaging (MRI) is highly effective in the diagnosis of myositis with regards to muscle atrophy. Short tau inversion recover (STIR) sequences are preferred to T2 sequences as fat increases T2 relaxation times
- New techniques include magnetic resonance spectroscopy (MRS), magnetic resonance diffusion techniques, magnetic resonance (MR) elastography, and idiopathic inflammatory myopathies (IIM)-related cardiac imaging.

Plain radiography

Plain radiography is not useful to evaluate the muscles of patients with myositis, except for detecting soft tissue calcifications. Chest X-rays may detect interstitial lung disease, although their sensitivity is lower than that of CT.

Videofluoroscopy evaluates the anatomy and physiology of the oral, pharyngeal, and oesophageal phases of deglutition. Videofluoroscopic findings of patients with dysphagia include signs of impaired propulsion (repetitive swallowing, residues in the valleculae, or piriformis sinus and crycopharyngeal sphincter dysfunction), as well as aspiration (Cox et al. 2009).

Computed tomography

CT has limited soft-tissue contrast, which hampers its capacity to detect muscle changes such as oedema. For this reason, CT has been supplanted by MRI.

Ultrasonography

Grey-scale ultrasonography

Grey-scale ultrasonography is best performed with a broadband linear-phased array probe with a 5–10 MHz frequency. The relaxed normal muscle is hypoechoic, with a speckled appearance in the transverse and a pennate appearance in the longitudinal plane. Ultrasonography can demonstrate muscle atrophy, fat, and fibrous muscle replacement and oedema, which manifest as increased echogenicity. Sensitivity of ultrasonography for myositis ranges from 2–82% (Pillen 2008).

Contrast-enhanced ultrasonography

Contrast-enhanced ultrasonography reveals increased muscle vascularity (Figure 14.1), a surrogate marker of inflammation. Blood flow and peak vascularity scores are higher in polymyositis (PM) and dermatomyositis (DM) than in controls, but with considerable overlap, and show poor correlation with disease activity (Weber et al. 2006).

Magnetic resonance imaging

Normal muscle

In healthy individuals, on T1 sequences fat and bone marrow are of high signal intensity, and cortical bone of low signal intensity. The muscle is of intermediate signal intensity, slightly higher than that of water on T1 sequences and much lower than that of water or fat on T2 sequences (May et al. 2000). Oedema, fat replacement, and muscle atrophy are typically absent.

Role of MRI in the diagnosis of myositis

MRI muscle oedema is typically found in 76–97% of active myositis (Fraser et al. 1991; Maurer and Walker 2015) (Figure 14.2A). Muscle oedema reflects water content (May et al. 2000) and is thought to represent active inflammation, although muscle oedema per se is non-specific and can also be due to intensive muscle exertion, infection, subacute denervation, ischaemia, muscle injury, neoplasm,

R   L

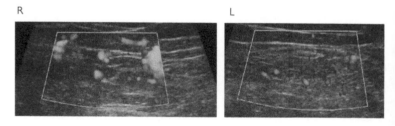

Figure 14.1 Increased vascularity (white spots) at contrast-enhanced ultrasonography of the thigh muscles a patient with active myositis. Exam performed with a Siemens (Antares) machine fitted with a 5–13 mHz linear probe after contrast (SonoVue®) bolus injection at 20° after 20' rest.

Images courtesy of Dr P. Macchioni, Rheumatology, Reggio Emilia.

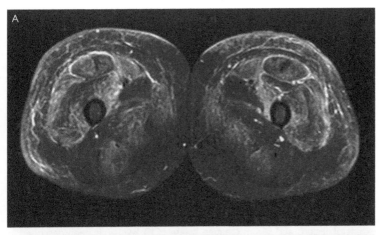

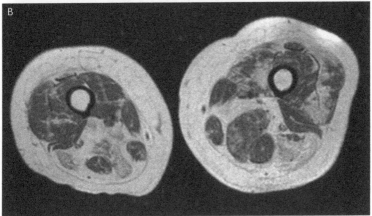

Figure 14.2 Diffuse muscle oedema in a patient with active myositis at MRI STIR (A). Fat replacement of muscle, more prominent in the posterior compartment, in a patient with longstanding myositis on T1 sequences (B) (both images: axial views of thigh muscles).

radiation therapy, and compartment syndrome (May et al. 2000). In myositis, muscle oedema is usually diffuse, although in juvenile dermatomyositis a patchy involvement has also been observed. Oedema can, in addition to the muscle, also involve the skin, subcutaneous tissue, and myofascial structures in DM. Oedema can be appreciated on both T2 and short tau inversion recovery (STIR) sequences as a bright signal within the affected muscles; STIR sequences are preferred because on T2 sequences fat results in longer T2 relaxation times (producing a bright signal similar to that of oedema), whereas in STIR sequences the fat signal is suppressed (Maurer and Walker 2015). Alternatively, fat-corrected T2 sequences may be used. Enhanced T1 sequences are also able to reveal muscle inflammation, but they are not superior to STIR sequences. Biopsying a muscle that shows oedema increases the bioptic yield. In a study, in which MRI was performed in 14 out of 25 patients with suspected myositis, only one MRI-targeted muscle biopsy was falsely negative, compared with five randomly targeted biopsies.

MRI can also be used to assess muscle damage. Findings of muscle damage are fat replacement of muscle tissue and muscle atrophy (Figure 14.2B), which are both best assessed on T1-weighted sequences (Maurer and Walker 2015). Like muscle oedema, fat infiltration, and muscle atrophy are not specific to myositis (May et al. 2000).

There is a limited correlation between MRI findings and other parameters of disease activity in myositis. A higher degree of inflammatory infiltrates at muscle biopsy has been linked to MRI oedema, while a fair correlation between MRI extent of lesions and serum creatine kinase (CK) levels has been described in myositis. Likewise, STIR intensity has been shown to correlate with physician's assessment of disease activity with a sensitivity of 89% and a specificity of 88% (Fraser et al. 1991). Combining MRI and muscle biopsy improves the diagnostic accuracy in myositis, decreasing the rate of false-negative results from 23 to 6%. When whole-body MRI is not available, MRI of the thighs is an acceptable alternative, since thigh muscles are virtually always involved in myositis.

Role of MRI in the differential diagnosis of myositis

MRI has been proposed as a useful tool for the differential diagnosis of myositis because different patterns of muscle involvement are observed in different myopathies. In DM and PM, proximal muscles are predominantly affected in a symmetrical fashion, although distal and/or asymmetrical involvement has occasionally also been described. The quadriceps femoris, the ileopsoas, and the pectineus are involved in approximately one-third of DM patients, but only exceptionally in PM. Compared with PM, patients with inclusion body myositis (IBM) show a more frequent involvement of the anterior thigh and of the distal muscles, an asymmetrical distribution, and more prominent fatty infiltration and atrophy. Muscle oedema is equally represented in both PM and IBM, but tends to be more frequent in PM patients as an isolated finding. In the lower limb muscles of IBM patients, there is preferential involvement of the quadriceps femoris, but relative sparing of the rectus femoris, while in the upper limbs the flexors digitorum profundi are typically affected. Overall, the diagnostic accuracy of MRI to detect IBM is 95–97% (Tasca et al. 2015).

In necrotizing, anti-signal recognition particle positive myopathy, thigh MRI usually demonstrates muscle oedema, particularly in the vastus lateralis, rectus femoris, biceps femoris, and adductor magnus with relative sparing of the vastus intermedius. Fatty infiltration is less common. The degree of muscle oedema here does not appear to correlate with serum CK levels.

- In statin-induced immune-mediated necrotizing myopathy, MRI of the thighs and legs shows muscle oedema in 62% and fatty lesions in 29% of patients. Oedema and fatty lesions are mostly found in the dorsal group of the thighs and superficial dorsal muscles of the legs.

- Chronic glucocorticoid therapy has been mapped to muscle atrophy and fatty infiltration.

- Many muscular dystrophies and congenital myopathies preferentially involve some muscle groups.

- Myositis ossificans is characterized by muscle oedema in the early stages before the typical calcifications develop.

- In acutely denervated muscles oedema develops 2–4 weeks after the injury. If innervation is not restored, atrophy with fat infiltration develops within months (May et al. 2000).

- Mass-like lesions are not seen in myositis, while they can be observed in neoplasms, abscesses, myonecrosis, traumata, myositis ossificans, focal myositis, and sarcoidosis (May et al. 2000).

- There is no specific MRI pattern for pyomyositis, where T2 and STIR images are both virtually always positive. On contrast-enhanced MRI, fluid collections show a non-enhancing central area and a well-defined enhancing peripheral rim. MRI is also able to depict involvement of adjacent structures when present.

Role of magnetic resonance imaging in the follow-up of patients with myositis

MRI is useful in distinguishing active myositis, characterized by muscle oedema, from chronic damage, characterized by muscle atrophy, fat replacement, or both.

In patients followed up serially, increased STIR signal intensity correlates with disease activity and return towards normal following successful therapy (Fraser et al. 1991). Improvement in MRI inflammation may lag up to two months behind clinical-laboratory response.

There is a validated MRI-based muscle- and soft-tissue oedema score for patients with juvenile dermatomyositis (JDM), but not for patients with adult myositis.

Scintigraphy

There is increased ^{99m}technetium pyrophosphate uptake by affected muscles in myositis, but also in other myopathies. The sensitivity of scintigraphy of myositis ranges from 50% to 100% (Buchpiguel et al. 1991; Walker et al. 2007). In a large cohort, sensitivity was 50% for biopsy-proven myositis, but only 36% of patients had muscle weakness and only 45% had a raised CK, suggesting that many patients had inactive disease, which can account for the relatively low rate of positive scintigraphy in this study (Walker et al. 2007). In contrast, in a study where all patients had a raised CK sensitivity of scintigraphy was 100% (Buchpiguel et al. 1991). Therefore, the main problem with scintigraphy in myositis seems to be its low specificity, rather than a low sensitivity.

¹⁸F-Fluorodeoxyglucose positron emission tomography

Positron emission tomography (PET) detects increased uptake of a fluorine-labelled glucose analogue (FDG) by metabolically active cells at sites of neoplasm, infection, and inflammation. In myositis, PET is mainly used to screen patients for neoplasms, but PET is also able to demonstrate increased FDG muscle uptake, which is usually diffuse and predominant in proximal muscles in active myositis Figure 14.3. The sensitivity of PET for active myositis was 33% in a study (Owada

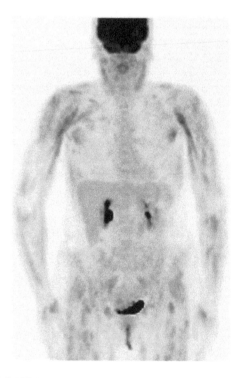

Figure 14.3 FDG PET (coronal view, maximum intensity projection) showing diffuse, symmetrical muscle uptake more prominent in the proximal upper limbs. Note the "arms down" position used to better visualize the upper limb muscles.
Image courtesy of Dr A. Versari, Nuclear Medicine, Reggio Emilia.

et al. 2012) and 75% in another (Pipitone et al. 2012). In the study that reported a 33% sensitivity, FDG muscle uptake was considered abnormal if it was greater than liver uptake. In contrast, in the study that found a 75% sensitivity the ratio of the average FDG proximal muscle to liver maximum standardized uptake value was determined in myositis patients and controls, and a cut-off value was chosen that best discriminated patients from controls (Pipitone et al. 2012). PET is highly specific for discriminating between patients with myositis from unaffected controls, but discriminates only poorly between patients with myositis and those with other myopathies.

Newer techniques

Magnetic resonance spectroscopy

MRS allows the presence and concentration of various metabolites within tissues to be determined. In myositis, indices of muscle oxidative metabolism are impaired, including adenosine triphosphate, phosphocreatine, and the ratio of inorganic phosphate to phosphocreatine. MRS is of value in monitoring patients with myositis, although the correlation with MRI findings is inconsistent (Cea et al. 2002).

Magnetic resonance diffusion techniques

Diffusion-weighted sequences measure random Brownian motion of water molecules within tissues. The random motion of water protons contributes to the signal. In inflamed muscles, there is increased diffusion of water molecules, which results in apparent diffusion coefficients being significantly larger than those that of unaffected muscles. Diffusion techniques may also provide abnormal signal in other conditions characterized by increased water content such as acute denervation (Baur and Reiser 2000).

MR elastography

MR elastography assesses the mechanical properties of tissue. In patients with myositis, there is a significant reduction in muscle stiffness relative to unaffected controls in relaxed state, arguably as a result of a significant destruction of passive structures or elements, like collagens within the muscle (McCullough et al. 2011).

Idiopathic inflammatory myopathies -related cardiac imaging

MRI has been used to investigate myocarditis in patients with myositis. Myocarditis is usually diagnosed when at least two of the following three MRI abnormalities are present: myocardial oedema on T2-weighted sequences with a signal intensity greater than two between myocardium and skeletal muscle, capillary leak (increased signal intensity greater than four between myocardium and skeletal muscle), and fibrosis, which is assessed on late gadolinium enhancement (LGE) sequences (Friedrich et al. 2009). On the other hand, myocardial LGE reflects acute cell injury, but may also reflect post-inflammatory fibrosis. MRI is more sensitive than myocardial scintigraphy and echocardiography in revealing the extent and site of inflammation, and its sequelae (Friedrich et al. 2009). After treatment with glucocorticoids and immunosuppressants, myocardial contrast enhancement on MRI significantly decreases.

Conclusions

Imaging procedures play a key role in the diagnosis and monitoring of treatment of patients with myositis. Muscle MRI remains the most important technique to assess degree and change of muscle inflammation and damage.

REFERENCES

Baur A, Reiser MF (2000). Diffusion-weighted imaging of the musculoskeletal system in humans. *Skeletal Radiol*; **29**: 555–62.

Buchpiguel CA, Roizenblatt S, Lucena-Fernandes MF et al. (1991). Radioisotopic assessment of peripheral and cardiac muscle involvement and dysfunction in polymyositis/dermatomyositis. *J Rheumatol*; **18**: 1359–63.

Cea G, Bendahan D, Manners D et al. (2002). Reduced oxidative phosphorylation and proton efflux suggest reduced capillary blood supply in skeletal muscle of patients with dermatomyositis and polymyositis: a quantitative 31P-magnetic resonance spectroscopy and MRI study. *Brain*; **125**: 1635–45.

Cox FM, Verschuuren JJ, Verbist BM, Niks EH, Wintzen AR, Badrising UA. (2009). Detecting dysphagia in inclusion body myositis. *J Neurol*; **256**: 2009–13.

Fraser DD, Frank JA, Dalakas M, Miller FW, Hicks JE, Plotz P. (1991). Magnetic resonance imaging in the idiopathic inflammatory myopathies. *J Rheumatol*; **18**: 1693–700.

Friedrich MG, Sechtem U, Schulz-Menger J, et al. (2009). Cardiovascular magnetic resonance in myocarditis: a JACC White Paper. *J Am Coll Cardiol*; **53**: 1475–87.

Maurer B, Walker UA. (2015). Role of MRI in diagnosis and management of idiopathic inflammatory myopathies. *Curr Rheumatol Rep*; **17**: 67.

May DA, Disler DG, Jones EA, Balkissoon AA, Manaster BJ. (2000). Abnormal signal intensity in skeletal muscle at MR imaging: patterns, pearls, and pitfalls. *Radiographics*; **20**: S295–315.

McCullough MB, Domire ZJ, Reed AM et al. (2011). Evaluation of muscles affected by myositis using magnetic resonance elastography. *Muscle Nerve*; **43**: 585–90.

Owada T, Maezawa R, Kurasawa K, Okada H, Arai S, Fukuda T. (2012). Detection of inflammatory lesions by f-18 fluorodeoxyglucose positron emission tomography in patients with polymyositis and dermatomyositis. *J Rheumatol*; **39**: 1659–65.

Pillen S, Arts IM, Zwarts MJ. (2008). Muscle ultrasound in neuromuscular disorders. *Muscle Nerve*; **37**: 679–93.

Pipitone N, Versari A, Zuccoli G, et al. (2012). 18F-fluorodeoxyglucose positron emission tomography for the assessment of myositis: a case series. *Clin Exp Rheumatol*; **30**: 570–3.

Tasca G, Monforte M, De FC, Kley RA, Ricci E, Mirabella M. (2015). Magnetic resonance imaging pattern recognition in sporadic inclusion-body myositis. *Muscle Nerve*; **52**: 956–62.

Weber MA, Jappe U, Essig M et al. (2006). Contrast-enhanced ultrasound in dermatomyositis- and polymyositis. *J Neurol*; **253**: 1625–32.

Walker UA, Garve K, Brink I, Miehle N, Peter HH, Kelly T: (2007). 99mTechnetium pyrophosphate scintigraphy in the detection of skeletal muscle disease. *Clin Rheumatol*; **26**: 1119–22.

CHAPTER 15

Neurophysiology in the assessment of inflammatory myopathies

Ranjit Ramdass

KEY POINTS

- Neurophysiology can play an important role in investigating a patient suspected to have inflammatory muscle disease
- The classic electromyographic abnormalities in inflammatory muscle disease include the presence of abnormal muscle fibre potentials at rest (fibrillations/positive sharp waves), early recruitment of abnormally brief and polyphasic motor units on volition, and relatively full interference patterns in clinically weak muscles
- Neurophysiological abnormalities can help qualify the severity and extent of disease, and rule out other nerve and muscle disorders that can mimic myositis
- EMG findings can help target an appropriate muscle for biopsy
- Neurophysiology may also be useful in monitoring treatment responses and to help differentiate between emerging steroid myopathy versus of a recurrence of myositis.

The electrodiagnostic examination

Clinical neurophysiology is essentially an extension of the clinical neurological examination. Electrodiagnostic testing should always be preceded by a detailed history and clinical examination, to help define the clinical syndrome and direct ensuing electrodiagnostic examinations. While standard operating protocols exist for performing electrodiagnostic examinations, an experienced electrodiagnostician will usually perform a targeted study in accordance with the individual clinical picture.

A typical electrodiagnostic assessment will generally start with nerve conduction studies (NCS), followed by needle electromyography (EMG).

The electrical properties and excitability of nerve and muscle fibres form the underlying basis for electrodiagnostic assessment. NCS are performed by non-invasive, i.e. surface, electrical stimulation of sensory and motor nerves, and subsequent recording of the generated action potentials. EMG is performed by the insertion of needle electrodes into muscles, and the recording of electrical activity at rest and during varying levels of voluntary muscle contraction. The generated signals can be amplified and displayed on a computer screen with appropriate software. Importantly, muscle electrical signals can also be transformed in to an audio output and differing EMG signals have differing associated audio characteristics. The combination of visual and sound-based assessment plays an important role in the identification and classification of the muscle electrical signal output.

Electrodiagnostic testing is generally well tolerated by most individuals, but occasional patients find nerve stimulation, or needle examination, uncomfortable or even intolerable. Although significant side effects are rare, needle EMG can cause bruising and has the potential to cause bleeding into muscles in individuals with bleeding disorders or on treatment with anticoagulant or antiplatelet medications.

Nerve conduction studies

A detailed discussion about NCS and peripheral neuropathy is beyond the scope of this chapter, and the reader is referred to more extensive texts (Daube 1991; Preston and Shapiro 2005). NCS are performed by artificially stimulating sensory and motor nerves, which are physically accessible to surface electrical stimulation (generally in the limbs), the responses being recorded by means of surface electrodes. In the assessment of a patient suspected of having a primary myopathy, at least one motor and sensory nerve in the upper and lower limbs must be tested to ensure there is no coexisting subclinical peripheral neuropathy.

Sensory nerves are tested by electrically stimulating the skin overlying sensory nerves and recording the induced sensory nerve action potential (SNAP). Commonly tested sensory nerves include the median, ulnar, and superficial radial nerves in the upper limb, and the sural and superficial peroneal nerves in the lower limb. Motor nerves are tested by electrically stimulating individual motor nerves via the overlying skin, and quantitatively recording the twitch induced in a peripheral muscle (the compound muscle action potential, CMAP). Motor nerves can be surface stimulated at various sites along their course to calculate the conduction velocity or to diagnose failure of conduction across a segment of motor nerve (conduction block). Commonly tested motor nerves include the median, ulnar, and radial nerves in the upper limb, and the peroneal and tibial motor nerves in the lower limb.

Peripheral neuropathies are traditionally classified as either axonal or demyelinating in type, depending upon the pattern of electrophysiological abnormalities detected. Demyelinating neuropathies typically show significantly reduced conduction velocities and/or conduction blocks, while primary axonal neuropathies are characterized by reduced amplitudes of the CMAPs and SNAPs, in association with relatively preserved conduction velocities. The presence or absence of a peripheral neuropathy, the type of neuropathy detected and the distribution of the abnormalities (e.g. symmetrical, length dependent, or multifocal) provides important information to aid diagnosis.

Electromyography

Needle EMG is the most important part of the electrodiagnostic assessment in the assessment of a patient with a suspected myopathy, including myositis. The electrodiagnostician will take account of a patients' symptoms and signs to guide the optimal selection of muscles to be sampled.

The functional assessment of motor units within muscles forms the basis of EMG. A motor unit is the smallest functional element of muscle contraction, and consists of a single motor neuron and all the muscle fibres that it innervates. Motor units vary in the number of muscle fibres innervated by motor neurons from just a few fibres per neuron in the extraocular muscles, to several hundred in large anti-gravity lower limb muscles. A single motor unit contracts in an all or none fashion and the action potential recorded by the needle electrode is called the motor unit action potential (MUAP), This is a summation of the action potentials of all the muscle fibres of that single motor unit firing synchronously (Preston, Shapiro 2005). The MUAP is usually a biphasic or triphasic signal (Figure 15.1). Muscle fibres closest to the EMG needle contribute most to the signal obtained.

Needle electromyography technique

Needle EMG is performed in three stages.

1. At rest, to assess for spontaneous motor activity.
2. During mild contractions to assess MUAP morphology.
3. During increasing degrees of contraction, to assess recruitment levels, and firing and interference patterns.

Assessment of spontaneous motor activity

Normal muscle is electrically silent at rest, other than at the end-plate region where the needle electrode may pick up small action potentials at the end-plate called end-plate noise or activity. During the phase of needle insertion the needle picks up electrical activity from traumatized/disturbed muscle fibres, i.e. insertional activity. This generally lasts less than 300 ms after cessation of needle movement. Increased insertional activity is a non-specific abnormality, and may be seen in a variety of neurogenic and myopathic disorders. Types of abnormal spontaneous activity include:

Fibrillation potentials and positive sharp waves

These are abnormal spontaneous discharges occurring at muscle fibre level. Fibrillation potentials/positive sharp waves are brief, biphasic potentials generated by muscle fibres due to membrane instability. This may occur due to

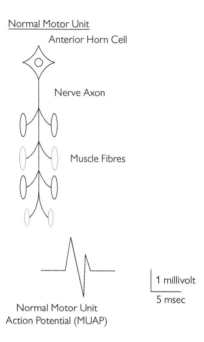

Figure 15.1 Normal motor unit and MUAP morphology. The normal motor unit action potential (MUAP) is a biphasic or triphasic signal representing the combined action potentials generated by all the contracting muscle fibres from one motor unit.

denervation or to muscle fibre pathology, including that from the inflammation component of myositis (Preston, Shapiro 2005; Daube 1991).

Myotonia

Electrical myotonia is the repetitive firing of muscle fibres. Myotonia has a highly characteristic output on the audio monitor, and sounding like a 'dive–bomber' or a motorcycle engine revving down. Myotonia is detectable in myotonic muscle disorders, such as myotonic dystrophy (DM1), proximal myotonic myopathy (PROMM), and myotonia congenita. However, electrical myotonia may also be detected in Pompe disease (GSD2), toxic myopathies, statin-associated necrotizing myopathy and sometimes in inflammatory myopathies.

Complex repetitive discharges

A complex repetitive discharge (CRD) is a repetitive discharge of individual or groups of muscle fibres with sudden onset and cessation, and may occur in a variety of chronic neurogenic and myopathic disorders.

Cramp discharges

Cramps are involuntary and usually painful contractions of muscle, which are electrically characterized by repetitive high frequency discharges of MUAPs on the EMG. Cramps may resemble the contractures associated with metabolic muscle disease, for example in McArdle disease (GSD5). However, contractures, unlike cramps, are electrically silent on EMG.

Fasciculations/neuromyotonia/myokymia

Abnormal spontaneous discharges that occur at motor unit level are markers of neurogenic disorders. Fasciculations are individual discharges of MUAPs seen in association with a variety of neurogenic conditions such as motor neuron disease, neuropathies from various causes and radiculopathies. Normal muscles can also occasionally exhibit fasciculations (i.e. benign fasciculations). Neuromyotonia is a high frequency MUAP discharge, which characteristically wanes in amplitude and frequency. Neuromyotonia is seen in peripheral nerve hyperexcitability states, such as Isaac's syndrome, but it is not seen in myositis. Myokymia is the repetitive discharge of MUAPs occurring in bursts, characteristically seen in radiation injury to nerve/plexus, but also seen in inflammatory neuropathies and peripheral nerve syndromes with hyperexcitability.

Assessment during low level muscle contractions (motor unit action potential morphology)

During low level muscle contraction the inserted needle electrode will detect signals from a few motor units firing close to the recording area. If the position of the needle is adjusted a clear sharp potential can be recorded. During low level contractions smaller motor units with a lower threshold for depolarization and containing mostly Type 1 slow-twitch muscle fibres will initially fire. As the force of contraction is gradually increased, larger motor units with higher thresholds for depolarization and containing more fast-twitch Type 2 muscle fibres become recruited. The morphology of these MUAPs can be assessed in terms of amplitude, duration, shape (morphology), and firing pattern.

Amplitude

MUAP amplitude normally varies significantly both within and between muscles. Amplitude is a measure of the size and density of muscle fibres closest to the recording needle electrode. In neurogenic disorders, the initial process of denervation is often followed by a regenerative process whereby healthy and still functioning motor units sprout new nerves to reinnervate the denervated muscle fibres. Muscle reinnervation thus results in larger motor units, and an increased amplitude of the MUAP. Conversely, in primary myopathic conditions including myositis, motor units lose muscle fibres resulting in lower amplitude MUAPs.

Duration

MUAP duration is dependent upon the number of muscle fibres within a motor unit and the dispersion of depolarization of the individual muscle fibres. In myopathic disorders the loss of muscle fibres from motor units results in a reduced duration of individual MUAPs while in neurogenic disorders the gain of muscle fibres resulting from re-innervation and loss of synchronous firing results in an increased duration.

Shape

Normal MUAPs have two to four phases (baseline crossings) or turns (serrations without baseline crossing). An increase in the number of phases/turns of MUAPs is termed 'polyphasia'. Polyphasia is a measure of the synchronized firing of muscle fibres within a motor unit and is increased with a reduction of synchronous discharge of muscle fibres. Up to 10% of normal MUAPs may be polyphasic, but in certain muscles like the deltoid, 25% of MUAPs may be polyphasic. Increased proportions of polyphasic MUAPs may be seen in both neurogenic and myopathic disorders, due to a reduction of synchronization of the contraction of muscle fibres.

Assessment during increasing levels of contraction/forceful contraction (recruitment/firing and interference patterns)

Low level muscle contractions result from the activation of only a small number of motor units. When such muscle contractions are initiated, the needle electrode will pick up individual motor units firing repeatedly at approximately 4–6 Hz. In normal muscle, as the force of contraction is increased, individual motor units increase their rate of firing (*firing pattern*) to around 10 Hz before other motor units are recruited. As the force of voluntary contraction increases further, more motor units are progressively recruited (*recruitment pattern*), and fire at progressively faster frequencies. This results in an overlapping and blurring of individual motor units on the screen (the *interference pattern*). In myopathic disorders, loss of muscle fibres within a motor unit results in reduced force per unit and so more units have to be recruited for a given force of contraction to be generated, resulting in early recruitment of motor units. The early recruitment of many motor units results in relatively full interference patterns in weak muscles. On the other hand, in neurogenic disorders the loss of motor units due to axon-loss results in reduced recruitment with the remaining motor units having to fire at higher frequencies before new motor units are recruited. This resulting in higher firing rates of individual motor units and incomplete interference patterns.

Electromyography findings in myositis

Nerve conduction studies are generally normal unless there is a coexisting nerve pathology e.g. due to diabetes, vasculitis, or a paraneoplastic process, etc.

However, a mild axonal sensory neuropathy may be seen in up to one-third of patients with inclusion body myositis. EMG may demonstrate increased activity during needle insertion/movement. In late stage disease insertional activity may be decreased due to muscle fibrosis. Abnormal spontaneous activity in the form of fibrillations is a characteristic feature of active inflammatory myositis (Blijham et al. 2006). Positive sharp waves and occasionally complex repetitive discharges may also be detected. The amount of spontaneous activity is a useful indicator of ongoing disease activity and can guide treatment. However, it must be noted that changes indicative of muscle fibre irritability/instability may also be seen in toxic myopathies, infectious myopathies, myotonic muscle disorders, and in some metabolic myopathies/muscular dystrophies (Preston and Shapiro 2005).

Low level volitional contractions in myositis show small amplitude short duration, polyphasic MUAPs (so-called 'myopathic units'; Figure 15.2). With increasing levels of contraction, early recruitment at normal firing rates is seen with full interference pattern on maximal contraction. Most inflammatory myopathies

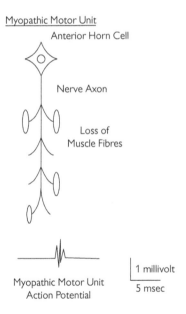

Figure 15.2 Myopathic motor unit action potential. MUAP morphology in myopathic disorders, including myositis. The loss of muscle fibres and reduction synchronization between contracting muscle fibres results in small amplitude, brief polyphasic motor units.

generally affect proximal muscles more severely, so these are sampled first. The paraspinal muscles may show isolated abnormalities and must always be assessed in suspected myositis. The distribution of EMG changes in IBM mirrors the clinical pattern of muscle involvement, with more prominent abnormalities detected in the forearm/finger flexors, quadriceps, and distal lower limb toe extensors (Joy et al. 1990). Reduced recruitment and rapid firing (neurogenic pattern) of motor units may be seen in late stage myositis, due to loss of muscle fibres or entire motor units. At times high amplitude, long duration polyphasic neurogenic type units may be seen with chronicity due to muscle splitting, regeneration, or hypertrophy rather than primary neurogenic involvement. Such neurogenic type units causing a so-called mixed myopathic-neurogenic pattern may be seen in one-third of patients with IBM (Joy et al. 1990).

In the classic work of Bohan and Peter the sensitivity of electrodiagnostic abnormalities was 89% (Bohan et al. 1977). EMG can at times be normal in milder cases, depending upon number and distribution of the muscles tested due to patchy involvement of muscle inflammation and resulting sampling bias.

EMG is useful for sampling a number of muscles in patients with mild weakness, and may provide information useful for choosing which muscle is targeted for biopsy. Patients may be able to compensate for mild weakness in large proximal muscles and EMG can reveal abnormalities in muscles thought to be clinically unaffected. The presence of unrelated abnormalities, such as neurogenic involvement due to coexisting radiculopathy, etc., can also be detected by EMG, and thus may influence biopsy site decisions. A muscle thought to be only mildly to moderately affected on EMG would be a preferred choice rather than one which is unaffected or showing end-stage changes.

EMG may also be useful in differentiating weakness due myositis relapse from that due to steroid myopathy. Recurrence of myositis is generally associated with prominent abnormal spontaneous activity (fibrillation potentials/positive sharp waves), while steroid myopathy is not associated with any significant EMG abnormalities (Buchthal 1970).

Neurophysiology plays an important role in the diagnosis of neuromuscular weakness and helps separate primary neurogenic disorders from muscle diseases in patients with similar clinical presentations. EMG can help qualify the extent and distribution of muscle disease in inflammatory myopathies, and can also help in the management and follow-up of these patients.

REFERENCES

Blijham PJ, Henqstman GJ, Hama-Amin AD et al. (2006). Needle electromygraphic findings in 98 patients with myositis. *Eur Neurol*; **55**: 183–8.

Bohan A, Peter JB, Bowman RL, Pearson CM. (1977). Computer-assisted analysis of 153 patients with polymyositis and dermatomyositis. *Medicine (Balt)*; **56**: 255.

Buchthal F. (1970). Electrophysiological abnormalities in metabolic myopathies and neuropathies. *Acta Neurol Scand*; **46**: 129.

Daube JR. (1991). AAEM minimonograph #11: Needle examination in clinical electromyography. *Muscle Nerve*; **14**: 685–700

Joy JL, Oh SJ, Baysal AI. (1990). Electrophysiological spectrum of inclusion body myositis. *Muscle Nerve*; **13**: 949–51.

Preston D, Shapiro B. (2005). Myopathy. In: Preston D, Shapiro B. (eds) *Electromyography and neuromuscular disorders*, 2nd edn. Philadelphia: Elsevier; pp. 575–89.

Outcome and treatment

Outcome assessment in the idiopathic inflammatory myopathies

Lisa G. Rider and Frederick W. Miller

KEY POINTS

- International consensus has been achieved on validated core set measures to assess myositis disease activity and disease damage.
- The core set activity measures were combined into validated consensus response criteria, which are recommended for use as clinical trial endpoints.
- Several other assessment tools, imaging studies, and biomarkers have been developed and partially validated to assess myositis disease activity and damage in all forms of myositis.
- Definitions of clinically inactive disease, complete clinical response, and remission have been proposed.

Assessing myositis activity

The idiopathic inflammatory myopathies (IIM), including adult and juvenile dermatomyositis (DM), polymyositis (PM), and inclusion body myositis (IBM), are rare autoimmune diseases that are characterized by chronic proximal muscle inflammation and weakness. DM patients have frequent cutaneous involvement, and all IIM have frequent extramuscular organ involvement. Given their rarity, few assessment tools and outcome measures have been validated for IIM disease activity and damage. Consequently, outcome assessments in past therapeutic trials used several different non-standardized measurements of muscle strength and function.

Recently, international collaborative groups, including the International Myositis Assessment and Clinical Studies Group (IMACS) and the Paediatric Rheumatology International Trials Organisation (PRINTO), defined consensus core set measures to assess myositis disease activity and damage in adults and children, then validated and standardized those measures (Miller et al. 2001; Ruperto et al. 2008; Rider et al. 2011). IMACS and PRINTO have also developed definitions of improvement that can be used as outcomes for therapeutic trials. These response criteria combine the core set activity measures to determine clinically meaningful improvement (Rider et al. 2004; Ruperto et al. 2010). Nonetheless, important gaps remain in the validation of these core set measures, and validation studies have yet to be performed in patients with IBM.

We review the major tools used to measure myositis disease activity, damage, complete clinical response, and remission, and discuss future trends in this area.

Measures of disease activity

Disease activity causes potentially reversible changes in anatomy, physiology, or function resulting from continuing inflammation in any organ system, changes which might respond to immunosuppressive treatments. IMACS and PRINTO have developed and validated core set disease activity measures, which are recommended for use in all clinical studies and trials to assess myositis outcomes (Table 16.1). These measures are most completely validated in juvenile DM (JDM), partially validated in adult DM/PM, and are occasionally used but infrequently validated in patients with IBM. Included in the core set measures of both IMACS and PRINTO are Physician and Patient Global Activity; a measure of muscle strength, as assessed by manual muscle testing (MMT) or the Childhood Myositis Assessment Scale (CMAS); and a measure of physical function, most commonly assessed by the (Childhood) Health Assessment Questionnaire. IMACS also includes the most abnormal serum muscle enzyme level and a measure of extramuscular activity, as assessed by the Myositis Disease Activity Assessment Tool. PRINTO, instead, includes a global tool, such as the Disease Activity Score, and a health-related quality-of-life measure, such as the Child Health Questionnaire. Many of these tools require training for optimal use, and suitable materials are available on the IMACS website (http://www.niehs.nih.gov/research/resources/imacs/diseaseactivity/index.cfm).

Table 16.2 summarizes other measures used to assess myositis in different subgroups, including additional measures of muscle strength and endurance (quantitative muscle testing and the Myositis Functional Index, an observational measure of muscle endurance and function); composite indices and functional scales for IBM; measures to assess cutaneous disease activity; and quality-of-life measures, such as the Short Form-36 questionnaire (Rider et al. 2011; Rose 2013). These additional measures, described elsewhere (Rider et al. 2011; Benveniste and Rider 2016), have been partially validated in subgroups of IIM patients and might be valuable in assessing function and organ-specific complications (such as interstitial lung disease or quality of life).

Imaging of muscle via magnetic resonance imaging (MRI) to examine short tau inversion recovery (STIR) or T2 signal (Schiffenbauer 2014; Maurer and Walker 2015), ultrasound to examine muscle echo intensity, or MRI of target organs (such as cardiac MRI to assess myocarditis) can be helpful adjuncts for assessing myositis. In addition to serum muscle enzyme levels, other helpful adjuncts to assess disease activity include immunologic biomarkers, including cytokines, chemokines, lymphocyte flow cytometry, endothelial activation markers, and other markers (Rider and Miller 1995; Olazagasti et al. 2015).

Table 16.1 Core set measures of disease activity in myositis

Name of tool	Purpose/content	Scoring	Comments
Physician Global Activity[a,b]	Overall rating of myositis disease activity based on all available clinical and laboratory measures	0–10 cm VAS	Somewhat dependent on experience of the rater
Patient or Parent Global Activity[a,b]	Overall rating of myositis disease activity	0–10 cm VAS	Distinct from physician rating
Manual Muscle Testing (MMT)[a,b]	Measures muscle strength by applying pressure to muscle groups tested against gravity or through a range of motion for muscle groups with less than antigravity strength	Modified MRC or Kendall 0–10 scales used. A total score of 14 axial, proximal, and distal muscle groups tested bilaterally (range 0–240) or a shortened version of 8 muscle groups (MMT-8; range 0–80)	Requires training in administration of the test. Does not distinguish activity from damage. Patients with muscle atrophy might not be sensitive to change.
Health Assessment Questionnaire (HAQ)/ Childhood Health Assessment Questionnaire (CHAQ)[a,b]	Assesses physical function in eight domains of daily activities	Range 0–3	Brief and easy to use. Well validated in JDM; limited validity in adult DM/PM; no validity in IBM. Significant floor effect
Childhood Myositis Assessment Scale (CMAS)[a,b]	Assesses muscle strength, physical function, and endurance	Range 0–52	Specifically addresses endurance. Reduction in bias and non-completion due to observational nature. Good psychometric properties in JDM/JPM; not studied in adult IIM. Significant ceiling effect

continued >

Table 16.1 Core seat measures of disease activity in myositis (continued)

Name of tool	Purpose/content	Scoring	Comments
Myositis Disease Activity Assessment Tool (MDAAT)[a,b]	Assesses six extramuscular organs to produce a global extramuscular score and muscle score, which gives a total disease activity index score	For MYOACT organ system scores 0–10 cm VAS. For MDAAT, each item is scored 0 = not present; 1 = improving; 2 = the same; 3 = worse; 4 = new, and converted to organ system scores of A-E, based on the intention to treat.	Best validated in adult and juvenile DM/PM; not validated for IBM. Requires training. Scores depend on the experience of the rater.
Disease Activity Scale (DAS)[b]	A global tool to evaluate muscle and skin involvement	Range 0–20, with muscle and skin subscale scores	Validated in JDM, no other IIM subgroups. Simple to use after training. Some items also include damage.
Child Health Questionnaire (CHQ)[b]	Evaluate physical and psychosocial well-being in a health-related quality-of-life tool	Summary score and subscale scores	Limited validation in JDM. Computerized scoring and tool associated with licensure fee
Muscle enzymes[a]	The most abnormal serum muscle enzyme level among CK, LDH, aldolase, AST, and ALT	Enzyme value, adjusted to common upper limit of normal for a multi-centre study	Only most abnormal one is used, which often is not the CK level in patients with JDM or DM.

[a] Part of core set activity measures developed by IMACS.

[b] Part of Provisional American College of Rheumatology/European League Against Rheumatism core set activity measures developed by PRINTO.

Abbreviations: ALT, alanine transaminase; AST, aspartate aminotransferase; CK, creatine kinase; DM, dermatomyositis; IBM, inclusion body myositis; IIM, idiopathic inflammatory myopathies; IMACS, International Myositis Assessment and Clinical Studies Group; JDM, juvenile dermatomyositis; JPM, juvenile polymyositis; LDH, lactate dehydrogenase; MRC, Medical Research Council; PM, polymyositis; PRINTO, Paediatric Rheumatology International Trials Organisation; VAS, visual analogue scale.

Data sourced from Miller FW et al. Proposed preliminary core set measures for disease outcome assessment in adult and juvenile idiopathic inflammatory myopathies. *Rheumatology (Oxford)*; 2001; **40**: 1262-73; Ruperto N et al. The provisional Paediatric Rheumatology International Trials Organisation/American College of Rheumatology/European League Against Rheumatism Disease activity core set for the evaluation of response to therapy in juvenile dermatomyositis: a prospective validation study. *Arthritis Rheum*; 2008; **59**: 4–13; and Rider LG et al. Measures of adult and juvenile dermatomyositis, polymyositis, and inclusion body myositis, *Arthritis Care Res (Hoboken)*; 2011; **63**(Suppl. 11): S118–57.

Table 16.2 Summary of selected additional measures to assess disease activity in myositis

Name of tool	Purpose/content	Scoring	Comments
Quantitative Muscle Testing (QMT)	Measures amount of maximum isometric force using specialized equipment	Values for each muscle group depend on devices used. Typically measures 8 or 12 muscle groups; total individual score for megascore	Quantitative measure that might be sensitive to small changes in strength or in measuring mild weakness. Requires specialized training and special hardware and software. Patients must have at least antigravity strength to perform. Limited validation in IBM and adult DM/PM
Myositis Functional Index-2 (MFI-2)	Assesses dynamic muscle endurance in seven muscle groups. Observational functional test	Each muscle group is scored as the number of correctly performed repetitions, varying from 0–60 or 0–120.	Myositis-specific objective functional index, which measures muscle endurance and repetition. Limited validation studies in adult DM and PM, but used in a number of exercise trials. Measures an important concept, muscle endurance
Inclusion Body Myositis Functional Rating Scale (IBMFRS)	10-point disease-specific functional rating scale	10 items, each rated 0–4; add individual items for total score. 0 = several functional disabilities, 40 = no functional disability or normal function	Measures important elements of daily-life functions that are often affected by the disease. Quick, inexpensive, and easy to administer. IBM-specific measure, with some validation and good responsiveness

continued >

Table 16.2 Summary of selected additional measures to assess disease activity in myositis (continued)

Name of tool	Purpose/content	Scoring	Comments
Inclusion Body Myositis Weakness Composite Index (IWCI)	9-item scale combining evaluation of hand flexor and quadriceps strength, timed functional assessment of limb girdle and axial weakness, evaluation of walking and swallowing	Range 0–100	Construct and predictive validity established in a large IBM natural history study
Cutaneous Dermatomyositis Disease Area and Severity Index (CDASI)	Measures several key features of skin activity and damage in DM	Scores range from 0–100 for activity and 0–32 for damage	Measures important components of skin activity and damage. Psychometric properties sound. Partially validated in adult and juvenile DM, including amyopathic DM
Cutaneous Assessment Tool (CAT)	Assesses skin disease in both activity and damage domains	Activity score, range 0–96; Damage score, range 0–20	Comprehensive assessment of relevant cutaneous lesions, including activity and damage. Partially validated in juvenile and adult DM. Abbreviated tool is shorter, easier to use.
Short Form 36 (SF-36)	Assesses global health-related quality of life, functional health, and well-being	Score ranges from 0–100, with 0 indicating maximum disability	Limited experience and validation in adult DM/PM. Easily administered. Available in multiple languages, with extensive normative data

Abbreviations: DM, dermatomyositis; IBM, inclusion body myositis; PM, polymyositis.

Data sourced from Rider LG, Werth VP, Huber AM et al. Measures of adult and juvenile dermatomyositis, polymyositis, and inclusion body myositis, *Arthritis Care Res (Hoboken)*; 2011; **63**(Suppl. 11): S118–57. Rose MR. 188th ENMC International Workshop: Inclusion Body Myositis, 2–4 December 2011, Naarden, The Netherlands. *Neuromuscul Disord*; 2013; **23**: 1044–55.

Response criteria

Both IMACS and PRINTO developed preliminary definitions of improvement that combine the core set activity measures into categories of clinically meaningful improvement. These definitions were based on consensus achieved by expert myositis clinicians who rated patient profile data developed from natural history studies and clinical trials. The definitions of improvement that achieved consensus were then used to test the sensitivity and specificity of candidate response criteria. Both the IMACS and PRINTO preliminary definitions of improvement require three of six core set activity measures to improve by at least 20%, with no more than one or two worsening, and muscle strength specifically cannot worsen (Rider et al. 2004; Ruperto et al. 2010). These initial response criteria were used in several therapeutic trials.

The criteria were recently updated by use of conjoint analysis and continuous statistical methodologies to formulate new consensus response criteria that should be more sensitive to change. The new response criterion is a hybrid definition with a total improvement score ranging from 0 to 100, which establishes thresholds of minimal, moderate, and major improvement (Aggarwal et al. 2017; Rider et al. 2017). The new criterion also uses absolute percentage changes in the core set measures and differentially weights the core set measures in the total improvement score, with muscle strength weighted most heavily, Physician Global Activity second, and extramuscular activity third, based on the results of the conjoint analysis survey. The new criterion is identical for juvenile and adult DM/PM, except that higher thresholds of improvement are required in juveniles. Also, the IMACS and PRINTO core set measures will be integrated into a single response criterion (Rider et al. 2017). These response criteria are recommended for use as endpoints in therapeutic trials for patients with juvenile and adult DM/PM.

Inactive disease and remission

PRINTO developed validated criteria for inactive disease in JDM. The best combination of core set activity measures to classify a patient as having clinically inactive disease is at least three of four among the following: creatine kinase ≤150 U/L, CMAS ≥ 48 of 52, MMT-8 score ≥78 of 80, and Physician Global Activity ≤0.2 of 10 (Lazarevic et al. 2013). The recognition that skin activity or other extramuscular activity can contribute to ongoing disease activity suggests that a refinement to require the inclusion of Physician Global Activity score to define clinically inactive disease increases the predictive validity of these criteria. Through consensus-building methodology, IMACS defined the criteria for complete clinical response for all forms of myositis as a 6-month continuous period of no evidence of disease activity while still receiving myositis therapy and clinical remission as the same but while not receiving myositis therapy (Oddis et al. 2005).

Damage

In myositis, damage is defined as persistent or permanent change in anatomy, physiology, or function that develops due to previously active disease or to complications of therapy or other events (Miller et al. 2001). Damage is often, but not always, irreversible and cumulative, and it occurs in 63–90% of juvenile patients and in 97% of adult patients after a median of 6.8–16.8 years of follow-up from diagnosis (Rose 2013; Rider et al. 2009).

IMACS has developed and partially validated core set measures for damage in children and adults (http://www.niehs.nih.gov/research/resources/imacs/diseasedamage/index.cfm). These measures include patient/parent global assessment of disease damage, which is a 0–10-cm visual analogue scale (VAS) of overall assessment of all damage, and the Myositis Damage Index (MDI), which comprehensively assesses damage in 11 organ systems (muscle, skeletal, cutaneous, gastrointestinal, pulmonary, cardiovascular, peripheral vascular, endocrine, ocular, infection, malignancy, and other; Rider et al. 2009). The MDI was inspired by the Systemic Lupus International Collaborating Clinics/American College of Rheumatology Damage Index and is intended to be used in patients with adult or juvenile DM, PM, or IBM. The MDI includes a series of VASs to quantify damage severity in each organ system, which together constitute the MDI severity of damage scale. The MDI extent of damage score is the sum of all the manifestations in all organ systems. There are 35 items in children, 37 in adolescents, and 38 in adults. To receive a positive score, each item must be present for at least 6 months (or the pathology that led to the feature must have been present for at least 6 months) regardless of prior immunosuppressive or other therapy. Only items present since the date of diagnosis are included.

The following approaches have been used to assess damage in myositis, but they have not been fully validated: laboratory tests, such as serum creatinine (Rider and Miller 1995); imaging of muscle to assess atrophy and fatty infiltration (Maurer and Walker 2015; Schiffenbauer 2014), including muscle MRI with quantitative assessment of fat fraction on T1 imaging; quantitative muscle ultrasonography; and computed tomography–based muscle density assessment. In terms of fibrosis of other organs, assessments by cardiac MRI and high-resolution computed tomography of lung have not been fully validated.

REFERENCES

Aggarwal R, Rider LG, Ruperto N et al. (2017). 2016 American College of Rheumatology/European League Against Rheumatism criteria for minimal, moderate, and major clinical response in adult dermatomyositis and polymyositis: an International Myositis Assessment and Clinical Studies Group/Paediatric Rheumatology International Trials Organisation collaborative initiative. *Arthritis Rheumatol*; **69**: 898–910.

Benveniste O, Rider LG on behalf of the ENMC Myositis Outcomes Study Group (2016). 213th ENMC International workshop: Outcome measures and clinical trial readiness in idiopathic inflammatory myopathies, 18-20 September 2015, Heemskerk, The Netherlands. *Neuromuscul Disord*; **26**: 523–34.

Lazarevic D, Pistorio A, Palmisani E et al. (2013). The PRINTO criteria for clinically inactive disease in juvenile dermatomyositis. *Ann Rheum Dis*; **72**: 686–93.

Maurer B, Walker UA. (2015). Role of MRI in diagnosis and management of idiopathic inflammatory myopathies. *Curr Rheumatol Rep*; **17**: 67.

Miller FW, Rider LG, Chung YL et al. (2001). Proposed preliminary core set measures for disease outcome assessment in adult and juvenile idiopathic inflammatory myopathies. *Rheumatology (Oxford)*; **40**: 1262–73.

Oddis CV, Rider LG, Reed AM et al. (2005). International consensus guidelines for trials of therapies in the idiopathic inflammatory myopathies. *Arthritis Rheum*; **52**: 2607–15.

Olazagasti JM, Niewold TB, Reed AM. (2015). Immunological biomarkers in dermatomyositis. *Curr Rheumatol Rep*; **17**: 68.

Rider LG, Aggarwal R, Pistorio A et al. (2017). 2016 American College of Rheumatology/ European League Against Rheumatism criteria for minimal, moderate, and major clinical response in juvenile dermatomyositis: an International Myositis Assessment and Clinical Studies Group/Paediatric Rheumatology International Trials Organisation collaborative initiative. *Arthritis Rheumatol*; **69**: 911–23.

Rider LG, Giannini EH, Brunner HI et al. (2004). International consensus on preliminary definitions of improvement in adult and juvenile myositis. *Arthritis Rheum*; **50**: 2281–90.

Rider LG, Lachenbruch PA, Monroe JB et al. (2009). Damage extent and predictors in adult and juvenile dermatomyositis and polymyositis as determined with the myositis damage index. *Arthritis Rheum*; **60**: 3425–35.

Rider LG, Miller FW. (1995). Laboratory evaluation of the inflammatory myopathies. *Clin Diagn Lab Immunol*; **2**: 1–9.

Rider LG, Werth VP, Huber AM et al. (2011). Measures of adult and juvenile dermatomyositis, polymyositis, and inclusion body myositis: Physician and Patient/ Parent Global Activity, Manual Muscle Testing (MMT), Health Assessment Questionnaire (HAQ)/Childhood Health Assessment Questionnaire (C-HAQ), Childhood Myositis Assessment Scale (CMAS), Myositis Disease Activity Assessment Tool (MDAAT), Disease Activity Score (DAS), Short Form 36 (SF-36), Child Health Questionnaire (CHQ), Physician Global Damage, Myositis Damage Index (MDI), Quantitative Muscle Testing (QMT), Myositis Functional Index-2 (FI-2), Myositis Activities Profile (MAP), Inclusion Body Myositis Functional Rating Scale (IBMFRS), Cutaneous Dermatomyositis Disease Area and Severity Index (CDASI), Cutaneous Assessment Tool (CAT), Dermatomyositis Skin Severity Index (DSSI), Skindex, and Dermatology Life Quality Index (DLQI). *Arthritis Care Res*; **63**: S118–57.

Rose MR. (2013). 188th ENMC International Workshop: Inclusion Body Myositis, 2–4 December 2011, Naarden, The Netherlands. *Neuromuscul Disord*; **23**: 1044–55.

Ruperto N, Pistorio A, Ravelli A et al. (2010). The Pediatric Rheumatology International Trials Organization provisional criteria for the evaluation of response to therapy in juvenile dermatomyositis. *Arthritis Care Res*; **62**: 1533–41.

Ruperto N, Ravelli A, Pistorio A et al. (2008). The provisional Paediatric Rheumatology International Trials Organisation/American College of Rheumatology/European League Against Rheumatism Disease activity core set for the evaluation of response to therapy in juvenile dermatomyositis: a prospective validation study. *Arthritis Rheum*; **59**: 4–13.

Schiffenbauer A. (2014). Imaging: seeing muscle in new ways. *Curr Opin Rheumatol*; **26**: 712–16.

CHAPTER 16

CHAPTER 17

Treatment of the idiopathic inflammatory myopathies

Heřman Mann and Jiří Vencovský

KEY POINTS

- Multidisciplinary care should be provided to all IIM patients
- Pharmacotherapy is the cornerstone of disease management
- Exercise is recommended from early disease stages
- In the absence of expected treatment responses, always verify the diagnosis
- Disease subtypes are characterized by differences in treatment responses
- Inclusion body myositis is treatment resistant
- Extra-muscular organ involvement requires more aggressive treatment
- Treatment side effects should be carefully monitored and managed.

Introduction

Idiopathic inflammatory myopathies (IIM) treatment is challenging, as these disorders are rare, have heterogeneous clinical manifestations, and incompletely understood aetiopathogeneses. There have been few randomized controlled clinical trials (RCT), these often involving small patient numbers, so treatment strategies remain mostly empirical. Management of IIM should be multidisciplinary, and tailored to individual patient's clinical phenotype and disease activity. The goal is to improve muscle strength and suppress extra-muscular disease manifestations, while minimizing iatrogenic complications. The first step is to make a correct diagnosis. This may be difficult, since many other myopathies have clinical presentations similar to the IIM, and even the presence of inflammation on biopsy does not exclude other diagnoses. Absence of expected treatment responses should therefore always prompt a diagnostic review. The next step is assessing disease activity, since muscle weakness may be caused by active inflammatory disease or instead the result of irreversible disease-induced damage (i.e. fatty replacement and/or fibre atrophy). It is important to consider the presence of poor prognostic features that may direct drug selection and treatment strategy. Higher glucocorticoid doses or early introduction of second line immunosuppressants are warranted when initial disease is severe, initial therapeutic response to glucocorticoids is poor or initiation of treatment has been delayed. The presence of certain autoantibodies and clinical manifestations such as dysphagia, or lung or cardiac involvement are associated with worse prognoses, and require more aggressive management. Treatment success is measured by improvement in major disease manifestations, assessed by testing muscle strength, improvement in skin rash, and organ involvement. In clinical trials a more formal measurement of response is a prerequisite for uniform evaluation, and new criteria assessing clinical responses quantitatively have been assembled by international committees. These developments are discussed in other chapters in this handbook.

The cornerstone of disease management, with a possible exception of inclusion body myositis (IBM), is pharmacotherapy. Physical therapy and rehabilitation should, however, both begin early on in overall treatment. Cooperation with a pulmonologist is advisable in patients with associated lung disease. Speech therapy evaluations and aspiration prevention are vital for patients with pharyngeal and oesophageal involvements. Osteoporosis causes significant morbidity in patients with IIMs; so its prevention and treatment are important. Appropriate immunizations should be given prior to the initiation of immunosuppressive therapy and pneumocystis prophylaxis should be considered in patients receiving high dose glucocorticoids or other immunosuppressants. All patients should be offered counselling, and psychological and social work services support.

Initial treatment approach

Glucocorticoids

Despite the lack of data from RCTs, glucocorticoids remain the key element of IIM pharmacotherapy, either as monotherapy or in combination with other immunosuppressants (Postolova et al. 2016). The usual initial daily dose is 0.5–1 mg/kg of oral prednisone, or its equivalent, followed by a slow taper after 2–4 weeks and, guided by clinical response, with a goal of reaching a maintenance dose of 5–10 mg daily within 6–12 months. Rarely, glucocorticoids can be discontinued in some patients. Intravenous methylprednisolone pulses (500–1000 mg daily for 3–5 days) are reserved for patients with severe disease. High dose glucocorticoids are associated with a number of serious side effects including osteoporosis, avascular necrosis, steroid-induced myopathy, and increased infection risk. Uncontrolled trial data suggest that lower dose or alternate day therapy may be effective with lower side effect risks. Efficacy and safety of oral dexamethasone pulses (40 mg/day × 4 days every 4 weeks) was compared with prednisolone monotherapy in a double-blind trial in newly diagnosed cases (van de Vlekkert et al. 2010). No difference was apparent in a composite score of disease activity between groups, but the cumulative glucocorticoid dose and glucocorticoid-associated side effects were less problematic in the dexamethasone group, although time to relapse was shorter in the dexamethasone group.

Methotrexate

The prognosis of IIM is worse when effective therapy is delayed. In more than half of patients, glucocorticoids alone are not effective or must be tapered quickly due to side effects, therefore various immunosuppressive drugs should be added early (see Figure 17.1). Methotrexate is frequently used here, although recent controlled trials failed to show efficacy in adults. In patients with established disease, neither methotrexate nor ciclosporin(by themselves or in combination) improved clinical features in patients with incomplete glucocorticoid responses (Ibrahim et al. 2015). Similarly, methotrexate-naive IIM patients did not benefit from methotrexate co-prescribed with glucocorticoids during the first year of treatment (Tomasova Studynkova et al. 2014). Nevertheless, experience suggests that many adult patients show improvement on treatment combinations with methotrexate. The combination of prednisone with either ciclosporin or methotrexate appears more effective than prednisone alone in juvenile DM patients, with favourable safety profile and steroid-sparing effects (Ruperto et al. 2016). Methotrexate has also been used in patients with extra-muscular manifestations, including interstitial lung disease (ILD), which should not be considered a contraindication to its use.

Azathioprine

Azathioprine can be used alone or in combination with methotrexate. A prospective, double-blind clinical study did not show significant differences after 3 months between patients co-prescribed azathioprine and glucocorticoids compared to those on prednisone only, but the combination led to better functional outcomes and lower prednisolone requirements after 1 and 3 years (Bunch 1981). Oral methotrexate in combination with azathioprine was compared to intravenous methotrexate with folinic acid rescue. Both regimes showed some benefit, with a trend in favour of oral combination therapy. Azathioprine is started at 50 mg/day and gradually increased to 2–3 mg/kg/day; but it may take 6–8 months to provide benefit. Thiopurine methyltransferase testing should be undertaken before prescribing azathioprine, and lower doses or alternative therapy used in patients with low-intermediate activity levels.

Antimalarials

In patients with predominantly cutaneous DM, hydroxychloroquine 200–400 mg daily is the preferred initial therapy, although improved efficacy has been reported when used in combination with mepacrine.

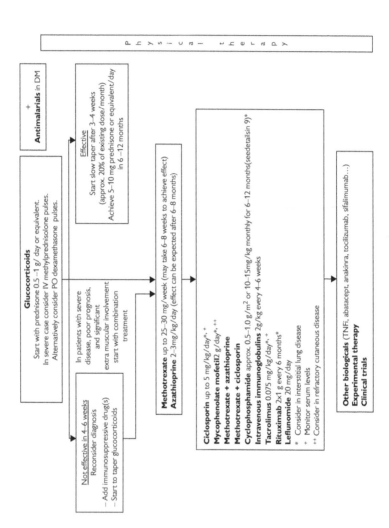

Glucocorticoids

Start with prednisone 0.5 –1 g/ day or equivalent.
In severe case consider IV methylprednisolone pulses.
Alternatively consider PO dexamethasone pulses.

Antimalarials in DM

In patients with severe disease, poor prognosis, and significant extra muscular involvement start with combination treatment

Not effective in 4–6 weeks
Reconsider diagnosis
– Add immunosuppressive drug(s)
– Start to taper glucocorticoids

Effective
Start slow taper after 3–4 weeks
(approx. 20% of existing dose/month)
Achieve 5–10 mg prednisone or equivalent/day
in 6 –12 months

Methotrexate up to 25–30 mg/ week (may take 6–8 weeks to achieve effect)
Azathioprine 2–3mg/kg/day (effect can be expected after 6–8 months)

Ciclosporin up to 5 mg/kg/day*, +
Mycophenolate mofetil2 g/ day*, ++
Methotrexate + azathioprine
Methotrexate + ciclosporin
Cyclophosphamide approx. 0.5–1.0 g/m² or 10–15mg/kg monthly for 6–12 months(seedetailsin 9)*
Intravenous immunoglobulins 2g/kg every 4–6 weeks
Tacrolimus 0.075 mg/kg/day*, +
Rituximab 2x1 g every 6 months*
Leflunomide 20 mg/day
 * Consider in interstitial lung disease
 + Monitor serum levels
 ++ Consider in refractory cutaneous disease

Other biologicals (TNFi, abatacept, anakinra, tocilizumab, sifalimumab…)
Experimental therapy
Clinical trials

Physical therapy

Figure 17.1 Treatment algorithm for adult DM/PM patients.

Approach to patients with poor prognosis or inadequate response to initial treatment

Ciclosporin

Some patients may benefit from the addition of ciclosporin to glucocorticoids. Ciclosporin was comparable to methotrexate in one study; however, a recent trial (Ibrahim et al. 2015) failed to show worthwhile effects either alone or in combination with methotrexate. Based on open label and retrospective studies, many experts advocate the use of ciclosporin particularly in patients with ILD and in the anti-Jo-1 positive anti-synthetase syndrome. We have encountered several patients resistant to other drugs, but who responded well to ciclosporin, maintaining long-term clinical responses even on very low doses.

Tacrolimus

Tacrolimus has been increasingly used in IIM, particularly in patients with ILD. Although the evidence is limited to small studies and case series, the results are encouraging. Small retrospective analyses of patients with PM/DM related ILD showed longer event and disease-free survival in the tacrolimus group (Kurita et al. 2015). A caveat is that regular blood monitoring, including of drug levels, is required.

Mycophenolate mofetil

Mycophenolate mofetil (MMF), used alone or in combination with other immuno-suppressants, has been found effective in the treatment of refractory PM/DM in a number of case reports/case series. When used with intravenous immuno-globulins, MMF was effective in severe and refractory myositis patients, with complete remission induced in all cases (Danieli et al. 2009). MMF has been successfully used in the treatment of IIM-ILD, including patients with amyopathic DM. A retrospective review of 50 juvenile DM patients MMF treated for 12 months showed significant improvements in skin and muscle disease activity, and a favourable steroid sparing effect.

Cyclophosphamide

Cyclophosphamide is effective in a variety of immune mediated diseases, although potential toxicity limit its use to that of a second line agent in IIM, and usually for patients with IIM-ILD. A systematic review of 178 cases (79% with ILD) treated in 12 mostly non-controlled trials and case series reported improvement of muscle strength and function, as well as favourable effect on ILD, in the majority of patients (Ge et al. 2015). Cyclophosphamide is usually administered as IV pulses in doses similar to those used to treat lupus nephritis or ANCA associated vasculitis. Long term remission induced by high-dose immuno-ablative cyclophosphamide dosage has been reported in a patient with treatment resistant immune-mediated necrotizing myopathy (IMNM). A potential risk for late malignancies associated with cyclophosphamide use is recognized.

Leflunomide

Leflunomide is a low-molecular weight synthetic inhibitor of T and B lympho-cyte proliferation, and approved for treatment of rheumatoid and psoriatic arth-ritis. Leflunomide, in combination with prednisone and/or methotrexate, was reported as effective in four cases of recalcitrant DM. Two cases of anti-Jo1 positive IIM-ILD were also successfully treated with leflunomide. Paradoxically, leflunomide may induce connective tissue diseases, including IIM.

Intravenous immunoglobulins

The efficacy of intravenous immunoglobulins (IVIGs) in DM treatment was estab-lished in a small RCT over 20 years ago (Dalakas et al. 1993). Subsequent trials were less conclusive, although IVIGs are considered as effective in some drug-resistant IIM cases. IVIGs may be used as a first line therapy in statin triggered IMNM patients with contraindications to glucocorticoids. IVIGs are also an alter-native for IIM patients with immunodeficiency, concurrent infection or in pregnant females. IVIGs are also potentially beneficial in the management of glucocorticoid resistant pharyngeal and oesophageal involvement. The standard dose of IVIG is 2 g/kg, divided in 2–5 consecutive daily doses administered once a month for 3–6 months. IVIGs may be used in combination with glucocorticoids and/or immunosuppressants. Subcutaneous administration was reported as effective for maintenance treatment after IVIGs, allowing for easier application and lower fluid overload risks.

Biologics

The most promising biologic agent for treating IIM is rituximab, a monoclonal antibody against the CD20 molecule and causing B cell depletion. Treatment tem-porarily removes B cells thatpotentially produce autoantibodies,are present in some inflammatory muscle infiltrates andparticipate in antigen presentation and interaction with T cells.

Early reports suggested effectiveness in about 80% of patients. The Rituximab In Myositis study involved 200 adult and juvenile myositis patients with insuffi-cient response to initial treatment with glucocorticoids and immunosuppressants. Patients were randomized to receive rituximab early (at weeks 0 and 1) or late (weeks 8 and 9; Oddis et al. 2013). The primary endpoint was not met in this study; i.e. there was no difference in median times to reach the definition of improvement (DOI). Secondary endpoints, which included 20% improvement in MMT and the proportion of patients achieving DOI at week 8, also did not dif-fer between the two treatment groups. However, 83% of randomized patients did meet the DOI by study end, which was better than expected in refractory patients. Treated subjects also reduced their glucocorticoid doses significantly. Eight out of nine patients who initially responded to rituximab and flared during the trial were successfully re-treated with rituximab. Seropositive (anti-Jo-1 and anti–Mi-2) patients improved faster than seronegative patients. Anti-Jo-1/Mi-2/

TIF1-gamma levels decreased and were correlated with disease activity changes; whereas anti-SRP levels were only associated with longitudinal muscle enzyme levels. Rituximab gave some benefit for IIM-ILD patients with anti-Jo-1 (Allenbach et al. 2015). The best outcome was seen in patients with disease duration of <12 months and/or acute onset/exacerbation of ILD in a retrospective analysis of 34 cases; six patients died from infection (Andersson et al. 2015).

Other biological drugs have hardly been studied. There is no convincing evidence for efficacy of TNF blocking drugs or anakinra, and there are several reports of myositis being possibly induced by TNF inhibitors. Efficacy of IL6 inhibition by tocilizumab was reported in a few cases, and a controlled trial is ongoing. A small study of abatacept suggested possible benefits in IIM patients. An increased type I interferon signature has repeatedly been described in DM patients, leading to a phase I trial with sifalimumab, an anti-IFN-alpha monoclonal autoantibody. The treatment was associated with suppression of the IFN signature in both serum and muscle of PM/DM patients, which positively correlated with MMT8 improvement; however, this study was not designed to evaluate drug efficacy. Despite individual case reports or case series reporting clinical improvement and/or steroid sparing effects in patients treated with biological drugs, these cannot currently be recommended for routine use.

Treatment of inclusion body myositis

IBM is characterized by progressive muscle weakness and wasting, associated with progressive dysphagia risk. IBM is resistant to immunosuppressive and immunomodulatory therapies. Some advocate trials of glucocorticoids and immunosuppressants, especially early on in younger patients, or those with rapid progression or with features of other autoimmune diseases. Given the questionable benefit of pharmacotherapy in IBM patients, careful monitoring of efficacy and toxicity is warranted, and treatment discontinued if side effects occur while symptoms progress.

Long-term IVIGs are not indicated for IBM. In patients with severe dysphagia some benefit was reported, although a recent Cochrane analysis evaluated the evidence for improvement as insufficient. A presumed role of T lymphocytes in the pathogenesis of IBM has raised interest in therapeutic exploitation of T cell depletion. Six patients experienced mild improvement of muscle strength after 7 days of IV anti-T-lymphocyte immunoglobulin followed by 12 month methotrexate therapy in a RCT. Thirteen patients with biopsy-proven IBM experienced overall slowing of muscle weakness progression with four even gaining some strength after receiving alemtuzumab (anti CD52 monoclonal antibody) in a proof of concept trial (Dalakas et al. 2009).

The resistance of IBM to immunosuppressive and immunomodulatory drugs, and improving understanding of its pathogenesis, has resulted in several alternative therapeutic approaches. Administration of a synthetic testosterone analogue oxandrolone had a borderline significant effect in improving whole-body strength and a significant effect on upper-extremity strength in a pilot RCT of 19 patients. Activin type II receptors (ActRII) mediate the signalling downstream of the myostatin pathway, this inhibiting differentiation and growth of skeletal muscle. A single dose of bimagrumab (a monoclonal antibody against ActRII) resulted in an increased muscle mass and improvement in 6-minute walking distance in a small, 8-week, proof-of-concept RCT. However, a phase 2b/3 study with bimagrumab did not meet its primary endpoint.

Exercise

Historically, exercise was discouraged in IIM patients due to concerns that it might aggravate muscle inflammation. However, a number of studies have affirmed the safety and benefits of exercise in IIM patients, including those with active and recent onset disease (Alexanderson 2016). Several different exercise programs have been evaluated in adult patients. Exercise improves muscle function, aerobic conditioning, and quality of life in IIM patients. One study also showed that creatine supplementation significantly improved physical capacity over placebo in IIM patients undergoing resistive, moderate-intensity home exercises. Several trials have demonstrated anti-inflammatory effects of exercise on gene expression in muscle tissues, including up-regulation of genes related to capillary growth, mitochondrial biogenesis, protein synthesis, cytoskeletal remodelling, and muscle hypertrophy and down-regulation of genes related to inflammation/immune response, and ER-stress response in repeated muscle biopsies. High intensity exercise is required to increase muscle mass, so may not be feasible for many IIM patients. There is no evidence that exercise has deleterious effects on disease activity, though no formal guidelines regarding exercise in IIM are currently available. Exercise load and intensity should be tailored individually, and based on the degree of muscle impairment, fatigue, and disease activity. Comorbidities and concomitant medications also need to be taken into account when formulating exercise regimes.

Management of specific situations

Interstitial lung disease (ILD) associated with myositis has better prognosis than idiopathic pulmonary fibrosis. Treatment with calcineurin inhibitors, MMF, cyclophosphamide, or rituximab is often successful. Patients with anti-MDA5 antibodies usually have rapidly progressive ILD, and need to be treated as early and aggressively as possible.

Calcinosis is common in juvenile DM, occurring in approximately one third of patients. It is less frequent in adult DM, but represents a very difficult problem. Evidence is limited to open-label case studies and case series, but no therapy has to date provided evidence of efficacy. The reports include use of calcium channel blockers, warfarin, bisphosphonates, sodium thiosulfate, aluminium hydroxide, probenecid, colchicine as well as IVIGs, rituximab, abatacept, infliximab, and thalidomide.

Treatment of *cutaneous manifestation* in DM may occasionally prove difficult. Patients should avoid sun exposure. Topical glucocorticoids or tacrolimus may be beneficial. Antimalarials are usually prescribed to patients with skin involvement, sometimes in combination with aggressive systemic treatment using IVIGs, tacrolimus, MMF, or other immunosuppressants.

Dysphagia usually requires high dose glucocorticoids. IVIGs may lead to dysphagia improvement even in patients with IBM. Airway protection is of paramount importance until pharyngeal recovery occurs.

REFERENCES

Alexanderson H. (2016). Physical exercise as a treatment for adult and juvenile myositis. *J Intern Med*; **280**: 75–96.

Allenbach Y, Guiguet M, Rigolet A et al. (2015). Efficacy of rituximab in refractory inflammatory myopathies associated with anti- synthetase auto-antibodies: an open-label, phase II trial. *PLoS One*; **10**: e0133702.

Andersson H, Sem M, Lund MB et al. (2015). Long-term experience with rituximab in anti-synthetase syndrome-related interstitial lung disease. *Rheumatol (Oxf)*; **54**: 1420–8.

Bunch TW. (1981) Prednisone and azathioprine for polymyositis: long-term followup. *Arthritis Rheum*; **24**: 45–8.

Dalakas MC, Illa I, Dambrosia JM, et al. (1993). A controlled trial of high-dose intravenous immune globulin infusions as treatment for dermatomyositis. *N Engl J Med*; **329**: 1993–2000.

Dalakas MC, Rakocevic G, Schmidt J et al. (2009). Effect of alemtuzumab (CAMPATH 1-H) in patients with inclusion-body myositis. *Brain*; **132**: 1536–44.

Danieli MG, Calcabrini L, Calabrese V, Marchetti A, Logullo F, Gabrielli A (2009). Intravenous immunoglobulin as add on treatment with Mycophenolate mofetil in severe myositis. *Autoimmun Rev*; **9**: 124–7.

Ge Y, Peng Q, Zhang S, Zhou H, Lu X, Wang G (2015). Cyclophosphamide treatment for idiopathic inflammatory myopathies and related interstitial lung disease: a systematic review. *Clin Rheumatol*; **34**: 99–105.

Ibrahim F, Choy E, Gordon P, et al. (2015). Second-line agents in myositis: 1-year factorial trial of additional immunosuppression in patients who have partially responded to steroids. *Rheumatol (Oxf)*; **54**: 1050–5.

Kurita T, Yasuda S, Oba K et al. (2015). The efficacy of tacrolimus in patients with interstitial lung diseases complicated with polymyositis or dermatomyositis. *Rheumatol (Oxf)*; **54**: 39–44.

Oddis CV, Reed AM, Aggarwal R, et al. (2013). Rituximab in the treatment of refractory adult and juvenile dermatomyositis and adult polymyositis: a randomized, placebo-phase trial. *Arthritis Rheum*; **65**: 314–24.

Postolova A, Chen JK, Chung L. (2016). Corticosteroids in myositis and scleroderma. *Rheum Dis Clin North Am*; **42**: 103–18.

Ruperto N, Pistorio A, Oliveira S, et al. (2016). Prednisone versus prednisone plus ciclosporin versus prednisone plus methotrexate in new-onset juvenile dermatomyositis: a randomised trial. *Lancet*; **387**: 671–8.

Tomasova Studynkova J, Charvát F, Jarosová K, et al. (2014). A prospective, randomized, open-label, assessor-blind, multicentre study of efficacy and safety of combined treatment of methotrexate + glucocorticoids versus glucocorticoids alone in patients with polymyositis and dermatomyositis (Prometheus trial). *Ann Rheum Dis*; **73**: 171.

van de Vlekkert J, Hoogendijk JE, de Haan RJ, et al. (2010). Oral dexamethasone pulse therapy versus daily prednisolone in sub-acute onset myositis, a randomised clinical trial. *Neuromuscul Disord*; **20**: 382–9.

Index